ANATOMY

OF A

PATIENT

Reginald Harvey

Joy Strickland

Copyright © 2018 Reginald Harvey & Joy Strickland

All rights reserved.

ISBN: 1986696022
ISBN-13: 973-1986696029

CONTENTS

	Dedication	vi
	Acknowledgements	vii
	Foreword	ix
	PART I	
1	The Diagnosis	1
2	Granny	11
3	Mom	25
4	Miss Tread	39
5	Lizzie	53
6	Dad	65
7	Sandra	93
	PART II	
8	Discovery Begins	125
9	A Little Help from my Friends	137
10	Hawaii with Cassandra	173
11	My So-Called Love Life	189
12	Revelation	219
	Afterword	239
	About the Authors	259

DEDICATION

This memoir is dedicated to the ancestors of my great family. Remembering them and recounting their parables and musings, I am reacquainted with the grace of my great grandmother, my godmother, my mother, father, and sister, from whom I learned courage, self-determination, and purposeful living.

I have to include here "The Crew", an eclectic menagerie of friends whom I now recognize as my chosen family – (*Padma, Joy, Cassandra, Marvin, April, Ranjini, Sonja, Sean,* and *Nedra P.*). These very special friends threw their arms around me as I began this chilling journey, and with love stood me on my feet.

> "A friend is someone to whom one may pour all contents of the heart;
> chaff and grain alike...
> knowing that the gentlest of hands will catch them – sift them...
> keep that which is worth keeping...
> and with the kindest of breath, blow the rest away."
>
> *-- Anonymous Native-American Proverb*

ACKNOWLEDGEMENTS

> "It's okay to burn the candle at both ends,
> but you can't have both ends lit at the same time!"
>
> -- Cora Luella Harvey (1918-1997)

Such was the sage advice my mother gave me when I started my engineering career at Dow Chemical USA – Texas Division. I was full of "piss and vinegar" and dead set on conquering the world as quickly as possible. Now, four decades later, I understand that she was counseling me to master the art of compartmentalization. She was telling me that it is perfectly fine to pursue multiple goals, but that to succeed, one must focus one's attention on one goal at a time. I would later come to understand the wisdom of separating *needs goals* (WHAT objectives must be achieved to survive) from *means goals* (HOW one employs skills and resources to achieve the NEEDS). Confusing the two may impede progress, and result in missed opportunities. Mom's wise counsel has become my cornerstone as I advocate for my survival.

I would be remiss if I did not extend my sincere gratitude to the incredibly knowledgeable and committed professionals who banded together to discover how best to save my life: my primary care physician, *Dr. Shahan Chowdhury*; my infectious disease specialist, *Dr. Claire Brennan*; and most notably, to my nephrologist, *Dr. Irfan Agha*.

A special recognition goes out to the men and women of *Methodist Dallas Health*

Center, The Kidney/Pancreas Transplant Center, The Liver Institute, and Texas Oncology Center, who embraced the peculiarities of my organ failure, and convinced me I could reach the other side.

I must also acknowledge my extended circle of care, those who have worked and laughed with me and scolded me for more than 40 years of professional and personal adventures. Although there are too many in this group to name individually, I must shout out to *Debbie and Tommy, Mark and Tina, Theodora, Carl, and JJ*.

Finally, I extend my deep appreciation to *Padma Min* who purchased Dragon Naturally Speaking in 2010 and told me I needed to write my story, and to *Joy Strickland* who helped me to do so, revealing to me the beauty in those mentors who nurtured my childhood, and shaped the man I would become.

FOREWORD

As a woman of East Indian heritage with many physicians in my family, my plan was NOT to be a doctor. Too much work. Too many years. But plans are meant to change. Not only have I become a doctor, but I've joined the ranks of a new breed of entrepreneurial physicians, bucking the fee-for-service model. My cohorts and I are known as concierge or direct patient care (DPC) physicians. We take care of our patients in a timely, effective, and efficient manner for a monthly fee – without the restrictions and rigid regulations of insurance. Why? Because we REALLY care.

I crossed the stage during my medical school graduation familiar with the concept of "directed learning", a pearl of wisdom imparted to me by one of my professors. However, only during my years practicing medicine, did I come to appreciate fully its meaning. "Directed learning" is the quest for meaningful and applicable knowledge, which drives me always to ask "why" – to understand the root cause of a problem or symptom – and never to be satisfied with a Band-Aid approach as I pursue the answer.

This way of practicing medicine allowed me time to hone my intuitive bone and understand what really makes sense when it comes to treating my patients. It was this intuition that landed me in hot water during Christmas 2015.

The story began as I sat at my desk disbelieving the low numbers staring back at me in siren red. All my members receive an annual physical exam with a basic panel of blood tests as part of their benefits. We drew Reggie's blood to lay a foundation for taking care of his health, but we had no idea we were opening a Pandora's Box. I picked up the phone immediately and dialed his number. Reggie didn't react as I explained his kidney function was very low. He simply agreed to drive back to my office and give another blood sample. Unfortunately, the second set of numbers was even lower. Now I was worried. How could this be? There were no clues in his medical history, and it was a Friday afternoon. What should I do? (Funny how these things always seem to happen on a Friday afternoon!)

I picked up the phone again and gave Reggie the bad news. I directed him to the ER. For what, exactly, I wasn't sure. All I knew was this new patient of mine had a kidney function that was unexpectedly poor. Once again, nothing disturbed his calm and steady demeanor. Although I knew he relished solitude during this festive season, he did precisely as I recommended. It was several months later, when I discovered how much he resented my direction. To this day, he reminds me of my Christmas season cruelty. In my defense, I desperately wanted to save him from the possible consequences of an undiagnosed issue, as he spent the holidays alone. Even though as his concierge physician, I was available to him 24 – 7 (just a text away), holiday medical coverage tends to be streamlined. I thought it best that he be under the watchful eyes of nurses and doctors during this time. Compounding the situation, I knew the on-call physician would ask, "So, why are you here?" And I thought Reggie might find this question unsettling and perhaps difficult to answer. Therefore, as soon as that call ended, I dialed the ER and requested the physician on duty. I don't remember who I spoke with, but I was somewhat embarrassed to say that my new patient had very poor kidney function, and I didn't know why. I asked, "Could you please begin the evaluation and get a consultant onboard during the holiday weekend?"

It was our good fortune that Dr. Agha, head of nephrology at the Dallas Methodist Kidney/Pancreas Transplant Center, drew the short straw to be on call for Christmas week. It was Dr. Agha who wanted to know why someone who looked healthy as Reggie was lying in a hospital bed, waiting to be seen. As he collected information from a multitude of sources, including blood tests, sonograms, and a kidney biopsy, the truth was revealed. Reggie was very sick. His kidneys refused to work properly after being attacked by several viruses, doing their quiet damage over many years. Who knew?

I truly believe in the adage, "you won't know, unless you look." The experience with Reggie and Dr. Agha has informed the way I evaluate my patients. I capture as much history as possible on the first visit, and compile a list of all possibilities. I then create another list of supporting blood and/or imaging tests: my wish list. With the advancements we have at our disposal nowadays, we can test for genetic outcomes as easily as we can test for strep. (I knew my undergraduate degree in genetics from University College London would come in handy one day.) As part of a new breed of practitioners, I pride myself in hunting for "pre-disease" – clues that predict the likelihood of a disease – and then working collaboratively and holistically for prevention. This approach allows my patients to understand their risks and engage proactively, investing time and effort toward improving their health. This is the work that brings me true joy.

Interestingly, I met Reggie through MC, my husband. Reggie was his colleague at CVS Health. Over a period months, MC shared Reggie's stories with me (many of which you will read and savor in this book). I found these narratives so compelling, I wanted to meet the person behind them. So the three of us met for dinner. I still remember that warm Dallas evening, sitting on the restaurant patio, working through the sushi menu. I was captivated by Reggie's purposeful and graceful mannerisms, his choice of words, and I love – loved – that he was a foodie. I live to eat. MC, on the other hand, eats to live. Reggie and I engaged in our banter as MC ate quietly. Remembering our time together, Reggie decided to try me as his primary care physician, after his long standing doctor passed away. And so began our fateful journey together on the road to Reggie's kidney transplant. Although the story is still unfolding, I have learned to value Reggie, not only as a concierge patient, but also as a friend and mentor. I feel in my heart that everyone is put in our path to teach us something. I have learned from him, that whatever happens, take a deep breath, meditate on the problem, and think clearly. A solution is bound to come. Then with a large glass of your adult beverage of choice and good gaggle of friends, laugh and make fun of all the things that could have derailed you, but didn't. You've survived another day to fight another fight, and you sure as hell enjoyed doing it.

I was completely captivated as I read Reggie's manuscript. The writing is both rhythmic and visual, projecting impressive images onto the screen of my mind, replaying so many of the stories I have delighted in hearing.

This is a journey of love, trust, and faith in yourself, your team, friends, and family... Enjoy!

Shahan Chowdhury, M.D.
Integrative Health and Heart
Integrative Skin ID
Frisco, Texas

PART I

1 THE DIAGNOSIS

It is Christmas Eve. No one knows I am in the hospital. I have been here since Monday. Today is Thursday. As the morning light from an overcast sky pours gently through the venetian blinds, I am bidding farewell to a jovial, middle-aged nurse who has gathered her belongings and is happily on her way home to her family. The door closes behind her as silence fills the cold, austere room like a ghostly presence seemingly conversant with these windows, doors, and walls, but alien to me.

Christmas is not my favorite holiday. In fact, Christmas is my *least* favorite holiday. Despite the ubiquitous Hallmark ads, I find Christmas to be the loneliest holiday of all. Everyone is either dutifully away visiting family or claiming a brief respite from relatives and the long-running and recurring pageants of competition, sibling rivalry, and insincere displays of Christmas cheer that go with them.

My family is dead. I have no one to visit or to avoid, so there is nothing at all unusual in finding myself alone, but to find myself alone *and* in a hospital bed is intense. I have yet to receive a diagnosis, and therefore cannot put my finger on the precise thing that warrants my unease.

My new primary care physician (PCP), Dr. Shahan Chowdhury, began to baseline my health profile in October after the death of my former PCP due to complications following surgery. As part of the profiling process, she ran a battery of tests and began to update my inoculations. A urine specimen taken last Thursday completed the process, but it was a show stopper. Protein showed up in my urine. Knowing that my vacation would begin the following Monday, Dr. Chowdhury contacted me, concerned that there was no clear explanation for the test result. She recommended a second opinion and instructed me to report to the emergency room at Baylor Scott and White Hospital for additional tests that would likely solve the mystery. At the hospital, it was decided I should stay overnight so that my system could be flushed with fluids prior to a second urinalysis. However, the mystery persisted, as the second test showed the same result as the first. The sonograms ordered Tuesday revealed cysts on my kidneys—a completely unexpected finding. As a barrage of questions concerning difficulty urinating, fatigue, loss of appetite, abdominal pain, jaundice, and other symptoms yielded no positive feedback from me, my case was referred to a specialist. Naturally, the hospital is on a holiday schedule, which means the availability of timely lab results necessary for a prompt diagnosis is compromised. As of Wednesday, the state of my health was still unknown. I underwent a biopsy to determine the extent to which the cysts may have damaged my kidneys.

Today I expect to consult with a kidney specialist who will discuss the biopsy results with me, and hopefully solve the mystery presented by the urinalyses. The hours creep by as I wait, existing in slow motion, while the world outside rushes by. I want to flee the cold and somber presence holding this room in its grasp, but there is nowhere to go—except within.

I think immediately of the nurse who is leaving the hospital seeking a moment of grace with her grandchild and I am glad for her.

I think mockingly of my vain attempt to make this Christmas a little different. I managed to arrange two weeks of vacation with no set plans to travel or attend any events. I set aside several thousand dollars just in case some unnamed opportunity for adventure presented itself. I was prepared to be spontaneous. Perhaps it is a good thing no such opportunity was forthcoming.

I think back on my family as I often do this time of the year. My parents passed away in 1997. My only sibling (an older sister) died in 2009 on Halloween. I did not know my paternal grandparents as they passed away long before I was born. I never met my maternal grandmother and do not know what became of her. I did get the chance to meet my maternal grandfather, Mr. Frank, one summer around my seventh birthday. I remember him taking me to the city pool for my swimming lessons. He would sit quietly in a lawn chair reading the newspaper with one watchful eye cast toward me in the pool. I don't recall any particular conversation with him, but I do remember feeling safe in his care, and happy he was present that summer. He died the following winter of a heart attack. I remember seeing the highways covered with ice as we attempted to drive from Waterloo, Iowa to Chicago for his funeral. The weather was so bad that my father arranged for us to continue the journey by train, which was fascinating. I don't remember feeling sad. Nor do I remember the funeral services. But I cherish the memory of him smiling at me from the side of the pool.

When I think of my family, I am reminded the holidays have not always been an exercise in solitude for me. There was a time when Christmas was magical. I see Iowa farmland covered with thick layers of wet snow and feel the crisp, cold air. I hear Irving Berlin's "White Christmas" playing on the car radio as we slip and slide down the highway toward my great-grandmother's farm. I am nestled in the back seat surrounded by mountains of blankets, expertly wrapped gifts, and delicious dishes prepared by my mother for dinner. I can't wait to reach that old farmhouse and see my great-grandmother's smiling face. I don't think much about Santa Claus. He is part of the holiday decorations, but he is not the focus of my joy. I anticipate hungrily the aromas inside the house, heavy with freshly baked cherry and apple pies, sweet plum dressing, turkey, duck, and homemade cranberry sauce, all mixed with the scent of the real pine Christmas tree decorated and standing tall in the parlor. I hear the creaking floors and the banter of adult conversation to which I'm not really supposed to be listening. My mother seems happier and more content here than she is in any other place. Years later I would come to understand why this is so, as I pieced together my mother's story and her relationship with this grand old lady. Soon enough I will be the center of attention, the object of my great-grandmother's hugs and kisses, and the audience for the wonderful tales she weaves about her childhood adventures on the farm. This festive occasion constructed of fantasy and reality lasts all day, an eternity for a six-year-old. I open my toys and nibble on cookies and slices of pie until I pass out for my afternoon nap. I awaken to dinner, followed by chocolate milk, more stories, and the chance to explore this two-story house that seems to go on and on and on forever. I am on a Lewis and Clark expedition, discovering a new world in every rung on every staircase and in every closet. My great-grandmother's home is a singular antique. Everything is in good repair, having lost none of its intended utility. I remember how so many handmade wonders—furnishings, handwoven rugs, linens, and draperies—came to life at the hands of this sweet old lady. She has lived on this land since 1866, and she has a wealth of anecdotes and witticisms that far exceed the limits of a child's comprehension. Still, I hang on eagerly to the sound of her voice and every word from her mouth. She and this farmhouse represent the magic of homestead and holiday joy. But Christmas magic ended for me with my great-grandmother's sudden death at the age of 101. It was in April 1967. I was twelve.

On the day of the funeral, I remember sitting on the front porch of the farmhouse, being comforted by the tender embrace of another special lady, my godmother, whom we all called Miss Tread. She was born in the late 1880's in the city of New Orleans. In many ways she is reminiscent of my great-grandmother, although she is some 20 years younger. On this solemn occasion Miss Tread senses my sadness and encourages me to take one last Lewis and Clark expedition through my great-grandmother's house. I enter with apprehension to explore the space. To my surprise none of the familiar aromas emanate from the kitchen or drift through the house. There is no scent at all and no hint of her presence. Although the furnishings are in place and nothing has been moved, it feels as if no one ever lived there. I return to Miss Tread's side and look up at her with questioning eyes. She simply says, "Granny is not there, is she?" Her words are followed by a gentle smile as she turns her head from me and nods slowly in the affirmative. "She is gone ... completely gone. She has left nothing behind as her work here is complete. Do not mourn her passing for she is in a much better place. She knows that we will all be okay." And with her words I understand Granny's essence has moved on somehow to another place, leaving behind indelible memories of those white Christmases I loved so dearly.

My reverie is interrupted as a slightly built figure enters the room, shattering the ominous silence like glass. He is crisp in appearance and looks directly into my eyes. "Mr. Harvey, my name is Dr. Irfan Agha. I am the nephrologist who reviewed your biopsy and I need to tell you that you are suffering from stage IV kidney failure. After reviewing the pathology I have determined that you suffer from both HIV and hepatitis B. These viruses have selectively attacked your kidneys for at least the past 15 years, rendering your kidney function below 15 percent. The lab has not yet reported viral loads, but I'm curious as to your awareness of these viruses."

My physical surroundings seem to shift instantly. I stare back at him blankly through the invisible wall between us. I wonder if I am actually in the same room as before. I struggle to digest what I just heard—but I feel I must say *something* for the invisible wall does not deflect the discomfort of his piercing eyes. I hear myself say, "I don't have HIV. And I am unaware that I have hepatitis B. You must have my case transposed with someone else's."

"No, Mr. Harvey, you *do* have both viruses and these are the reasons your kidney function is in the condition it is."

"That is impossible. I have been checked for HIV every year and told by my doctor that my system is clean."

"Our results are conclusive. Your condition is serious. You could have gone to sleep and never awakened. Again, these viruses have been in your system for at least 15 years, if not longer."

Dr. Agha stops speaking and stares at me as if perplexed. The awesome silence returns with a vengeance. Perhaps he is trying to determine whether the specter before him is deception or denial. I return his stare with utter disbelief. This has to be a bad joke, but neither of us is laughing. I want to escape from this place and go home. I try to figure out how I am going to get this madman to discharge me just as he breaks the silence to offer a reprieve, saying, "I have decided to let you go home this morning, but I want to see you in my office next week for outpatient evaluation. I strongly suggest you contact an infectious disease doctor as soon as possible. The hospital will provide you with contact information for the North Texas infectious disease referral system." With those words he pivots, swings the door open, and exits.

The silence returns, but this time it is easily dwarfed by my loneliness. I feel more alone than I have felt at any time in my entire life. I replay the scene over and over in my head in utter disbelief. I look around the inhospitable room and find my clothes stacked neatly on the radiator. I need to get dressed. I need to get out of here. I throw my legs over the side of the bed and stand up, realizing for the first time that I feel as though I weigh 500 pounds. As I struggle to cross the short distance from the bed to the radiator, I feel exhausted. I am confused. I just want to go home.

I begin to dress slowly, but fall back on the bed to regain my strength and ease the shock. I adjust to a sitting position and wait for my discharge papers. Another hour passes before a nurse enters the room to inform me that my paperwork is on its way. After another half-hour, the doctor on duty comes in, quickly reviews the notes on the discharge papers and leaves them for my signature. I am free to go.

I locate my car keys and tentatively walk toward the door. Once in the hallway, I focus on the signage to find the nearest exit. After wandering through a maze of hallways, I stumble upon an exterior door. Outside, I find I am disoriented. I search my mind frantically, trying to recall which parking garage holds my car. I walk to the corner and find a bench at a bus stop within the Baylor campus. I sit down to get my bearings and suddenly remember the GPS locator function on my cell phone. I can use this to locate my car with the vehicle app. I have never used the function before but I am desperate. I will figure it out. After several attempts I am able to determine that the garage I want is half a block away. I stand up and start walking. Once inside the garage, I activate the alarm to locate my car. I open the door and fall into the driver's seat. I sit there for what seems like another hour before I start the engine and drive toward the exit.

I don't remember much about the drive home. The car seems to know the way. Once parked, I rally all my strength to make my way to my condo. Inside, I collapse in my recliner and sit there alone, waiting quietly, immersed in the familiar silence of home.

I struggle to recall the days of the week. I remember starting my vacation in the emergency room Monday, but everything else is a blur. Christmas is tomorrow and this is not how I envisioned spending it. I am exhausted and lost in my thoughts. Suddenly Dr. Agha's voice bursts through the veil of my stupor, talking nonsense. "Mr. Harvey, your condition is serious... You could have gone to sleep and never awakened."

Did I really hear him say that or was I hallucinating? No. I remember. He said I could have fallen asleep and never awakened. And no one would have been the wiser—including me. How could this happen? I felt fine before checking into the hospital. In the past two years I adjusted my diet, began to work out regularly, and walk three miles every other day, despite maintaining a crazy, self-imposed work schedule: awake at 4:30 AM; in the office by 6:30; and back home at 6 p.m. I had been looking forward to this two-week vacation to recharge my battery. Now what? I can't explain this to myself; how could I possibly explain it to anyone else? The season of tacky Christmas songs, fake smiles, and senseless parties with too much food and alcohol has sunk to a new low, and is threatening to take me down with it.

I realize I have more questions than answers, and no idea what the prognosis may be for my future, if indeed I have a future. I want to stop thinking. Again I feel the extreme heaviness of my body as I struggle to lean back and raise my feet and legs, allowing my weight to be supported and embraced by the recliner. Dozing off and on, I suddenly awaken to the familiar aromas inside Granny's farmhouse. The air is again heavy with freshly baked cherry and apple pies, sweet plum dressing, turkey, duck, and homemade cranberry sauce, all mixed with the scent of the real pine Christmas tree decorated and standing tall in the parlor. I am startled to feel the gentle touch of Granny's hand stroking the back of my own. I am sitting at that familiar old ebony dining room table, surrounded by cookies and pies. Granny smiles at me with those piercing blue-gray eyes that hold me in a hypnotic gaze. She speaks and I hear her words, but her voice is the voice of my mother. Then I remember how the two of them spoke with such similar inflections and speech patterns…"Remember, when you sweep something under the rug, life will eventually pull back that rug and reveal the ugly mess that has festered in the dark. What's done in the dark will come to the light."

"Child, did you ever wonder how I managed to survive for a century? How I was born in the aftermath of the Civil War, and lived to see the civil rights movement?" I look at her sweet face, noticing for the first time that there are no wrinkles or crepey skin surrounding her eyes or mouth. Her skin seems to glow, emphasizing those signature high cheekbones. Her hands are strong from a century of hard work, yet they remain supple and smooth as she continues to stroke my hand gently.

"Will you have another slice of pie?" With her question, I open my eyes. I breathe deeply once, and then again. Despite mammoth uncertainty, a new awareness ushers in the first sense of peace I have felt in days. Is this my Christmas gift? Is this how it all ends? Or is this the dawn of a new beginning?

I close my eyes again, smiling this time, as I accept Granny's offer of another slice of pie.

2 Granny

Interlude

When Dr. Agha informed me that I could have gone to sleep and never awakened, I was shocked into the realization that in the preceding days, months, and years, I had been living on borrowed time. If ignorance is bliss, then surely knowledge can bring distress. Indeed, as I began to inhabit my life with this new knowledge, unhappiness was the common thread connecting the barrage of new terms, processes, and systems I was forced to navigate. My former identity as a competent and respected business professional with a vigorous work schedule, living life on my terms, was displaced with doctor visits, medical insurance claims, and the pursuit of life-saving pharmaceuticals. Reluctantly, I found it necessary to embrace my new identity as a *patient* – a patient fighting for my life. But a patient is first and foremost a *person* with a culture, racial identity, family history, beliefs, education, strengths, and weaknesses. Not only do these factors influence potentially how the patient is received by the health care system, but I believe they also bear heavily on how the patent engages the battle.

As an African American man, I am aware it is sometimes hard to know how race and other factors may complicate my life and compound the struggles I may face. I am the beneficiary of a rich and, in many ways, a difficult family history. Whether because of the difficulties or in spite of them, memories of the people who were most influential during my early years in Iowa, were always rambling around somewhere in my head. Even before my diagnosis, bits and pieces would spill out from time to time like fragments of a vase, once fine, but now broken. Without a shred of self-consciousness, I would share those fragments with anyone willing to listen. Speaking their names was enough to evoke their presence. They felt closer to me, alive even. After my diagnosis, my recall grew even more vivid and intense. Memories that began with Granny while I was still hospitalized, continued to flow and expand into feature-length films filled with images, sounds, and emotions, starring Miss Tread (my godmother) and Mom and Dad, with my sister Sandra, Lizzie, and others playing supporting roles. It was an early and entirely unexpected revelation that in the process of sharing this medical journey through the lens of my family history, I might find the strength, courage, and resolve I must summon as I engage in this fight for survival.

Still, it must be said that writing this book was not my own idea. Many years before my diagnosis, while pursuing my M.S. degree at the University Of Texas McCombs School Of Business, I met and developed a wonderful and lasting friendship with Padma, a fellow student. As we got to know each other and learn about our respective backgrounds, fragments of the vase would spill over into my conversations with her. After a while Padma began to urge me to write about the characters I shared. Although her pleas fell on deaf ears—for years—she gifted me eventually the Dragon dictation software as if to make her wishes manifest.

When I met Joy (my co-author) in 2009, she was leading the nonprofit organization she founded fifteen years earlier. We became fast friends in short order. In fact, I joined her organization's board of directors. Naturally, we often discussed our life experiences, and once again, fragments of my family history spilled out, becoming a mainstay of our conversations. Later, as I began to share with her the details of the bombshell diagnosis dropped on me the previous December, Joy began to echo the appeals I heard for so many years from Padma. I remained unconvinced, but Joy was even more persistent than Padma had been. She said, "Most people, especially African Americans, don't value their stories. They go through stuff—and they go on." Joy was unyielding in her belief that my story could be helpful and inspirational even, to others traversing the aftermath of a difficult diagnosis.

In time I began to contemplate gathering the fragments and piecing together the broken vase. Maybe someone *could* appreciate this uncertain and tenuous journey. And maybe I could give the amazing people who shaped my life, their due.

It was time to take the Dragon software off the shelf.

***

Granny

I shared briefly in the previous chapter some of my memories of Granny, my maternal great-grandmother, so I will continue here with her story.

Granny was born in Iowa in 1866 to a young couple who had been married off near the end of the Civil War. As the story goes, Granny's parents were born on two adjoining plantations in the South. The plantation owners fathered these children by their enslaved black women. The children looked too much like their white fathers, which prompted the plantation owners to "free" them, marry them off (to each other), and resettle them on 160 acres, which they acquired in Iowa coal country. When she came of age, Granny married a coal miner from Missouri, Robert Franklin (reported to have been of Dutch heritage) on October 13, 1887 in Kirkville, Iowa. Together they managed the farm when he was not away working the rich strip mines of Iowa and Missouri.

Granny gave birth to 17 children from 1888 to 1912, including (I am told) three sets of twins. I knew only five of Granny's children. There was Luella "Sister" Franklin, the oldest daughter (born July 1888), who was a very conservative and proper woman. Although I was aware of Jessie Franklin (born April 1891), for years I was uncertain of her connection to the family. I was always afraid of her because she looked like the Wicked Witch of the West in the 1936 classic movie/musical *The Wonderful Wizard of Oz*. Horace Franklin (born March 1893), my grandfather, apparently resembled his Dutch father in appearance, sporting wavy, dark blond hair, accentuated by blue-gray eyes and a strong square jaw. Rupert L Franklin (July 9, 1898 – July 28, 1994) became a very successful lawyer and relocated to Detroit, Michigan in the early 1940's. He was a dead ringer for singer Bing Crosby. Finally, there was Roberta "Bobbye" Franklin (born in 1912) who was only six years older than my mother.

Cora Llewelyn Franklin, my mother, was born July 6, 1918 in Ottumwa, Iowa to Horace Franklin, Jr. and his wife, the daughter of an Indian chief. I never knew my maternal grandmother's name or her tribe, although it was most likely descended from the prehistoric Oneota cultures who were Dakotan-Siouan speakers. Early in the twentieth century, these peoples were known as Osage, Ponca, Pawnee, and Sauk Indians or a tribal variation thereof. My mother's parents separated when she was only two years old, and later divorced. Her father had a reputation as a ladies' man, something his wife would have found intolerable, considering her culture and privileged heritage.

I remember a picture of Little Cora in a white, handmade dress with a high buttoned collar and leather calf-high laced boots. The fair-skinned little girl with tightly curled hair sat in a wooden chair next to her four-year-old brother, Jack, a handsome, dark-skinned little boy with silky black hair. After the divorce, Cora's mother returned to her tribe, but neither Cora nor her brother was allowed to become part of this community because they were of mixed blood (black, white, and Indian). At this point, *colorism* began to frame Little Cora's fate, and continued to have an impact on her life as an adult.

Colorism refers to prejudiced attitudes and discriminatory practices based on skin color. As a result of three centuries of American enslavement and Jim Crow laws predicated on white supremacy , it is widely held that African Americans suffer from internalized racism, accepting as truth our own inferiority, preferring European facial features, skin color, and culture to our own. Colorism is thought to be one of many symptoms of internalized racism. The rift that began on the plantation, continued during the Jim Crow era (from the late 1890's through the mid-1960's), and indeed, is still present today in some quarters.

Apparently, the Allen branch of the family (children of Granny's sisters and/or brothers) were dark-skinned, unlike Granny, who could "pass" for white. No one from this branch of the family would accept Little Cora because she was fair-skinned.

So Little Cora and Little Jack were separated. Jack went to live with the Allen branch of the family in Ames, Iowa, while Cora went to live with Granny, the woman after whom she was named, and the only person willing to take her in.

Granny lived where she was born, on the 160-acre farm in Oskaloosa, Iowa purchased by her grandfathers. And this would be Little Cora's new home. Oskaloosa was a farming community in Mahaska County, which was formally platted in 1844 by Nathan Boone, the youngest son of frontiersman Daniel Boone.

In the 1880's, more than one million tons of bituminous coal was mined in the area.

Little Cora's new home, like most farms, was a unique, organic and almost sentient thing. Every component followed the established engineering construct of *form, fit, and function*. No component was left idle. Everything—structures, tools, livestock, fields, and the people who lived and worked on the farm—must justify its existence.

The farmhouse was the epicenter, sheltering its inhabitants, providing the facilities for cooking and serving meals, and offering a rest and recuperation. Beneath the footprint of the farmhouse, the cellar was constructed of tightly packed earth for walls, and slightly less compacted earth on the floor. The walls remained moist and cool due to the natural settlement of rainwater. In summer, strategically placed registers allowed this cool, moist air to circulate from the cellar through the farmhouse. The cool, loosely compacted floor provided a suitable place for fermenting beer, except when the cellar overheated. At those times, glass bottles of brew buried in the cellar floor with only the bottleneck exposed, could explode like gunshots, blowing off the bottle caps.

Six to ten feet deep porches on the east, west, and south sides of the two-story farmhouse offered protection from winter's hard freezes, lasting from early November through late April. The east porch caught the early morning sun, the southern porch captured the wind, and the western porch shielded the hot afternoon radiant heat. The windows on each porch could be raised or lowered to shut out the elements or welcome them in.

In winter the windows of the Western porch captured the radiant heat and distributed it around the Southern and Eastern porches, which wrapped the house like a blanket, retaining the heat produced by an oil-fired furnace in the basement. In springtime the porches served as a transitional space between the hearth of the farmhouse and the thawing grounds outside. In summer the porches provided shade from the relentless sun and distributed a steady current of air around the exterior walls to cool the interior. And in fall, the porches provided an extended living space for napping, smoking, and drinking lemonade or homemade brew.

In spring, summer, and fall, the porches provided space where laundry could be hung to dry in the breezes, protected from rain. This function cannot be overstated. Today, laundry is an easy, thoughtless, and sometimes haphazard enterprise, but prior to World War II, doing laundry was a Herculean task. Even considering the myriad of responsibilities in Granny's purview, washday was surely the most laborious and time-consuming.

In preparation for washday, wood must be chopped and soap made. A huge cast-iron pot, two to three feet deep was central to the process. Washday began at sunrise and ended ten to twelve hours later.

The punch list was an extensive one. Chop wood for the fire pit. Set up the fire pit about fifteen feet from the house. Gather water to fill the cast-iron pot. Build a roaring fire beneath the pot. Bring the water to a boil. Use a wash stick (of hickory or oak) to churn dirty clothes in the hot soapy water, and lift and transfer them to a washtub filled with cold water. Manually rub the clothes up and down over a washboard to remove any remaining dirt and stains. Hand wring the washed clothes and set them aside. Empty the washtub and refill with water for a rinse cycle. Agitate clothes to remove soap. Hand wring each item to remove as much water as possible. Pour out rinse water and refill the wash tub as necessary to assure water is clean enough to remove soap from clothes. Carry the hand-wrung clothes to the close line, and attach each item using wooden clothes pins. Extinguish the fire. Empty both washtub and cast-iron pot.

Certain events on the evening of a particular washday are a standout in family lore.

Washday did not relieve Granny of other chores. If vegetables needed to be harvested, livestock dressed, or meals prepared, so be it. She did it. As was often the case, suppertime was delayed on this particular day because Grandpa Franklin arrived late from his work in the coal mines. He came in, cleaned himself up and assumed his place at the head of the table.

Everyone was seated at the same grand dining room table that fascinated me as a child. The table seated twelve comfortably, and could accommodate with ease an enormous banquet. The finish was dark, almost ebony. The massive turned legs with claw feet supported a table top about five inches thick.

There was an unwritten rule in the Franklin household that Grandpa Franklin always was served first. True to form, Granny dutifully set Grandpa Franklin's place and brought his bowl of stew and a beer. She then proceeded to serve her youngest daughter, Roberta, Little Cora (my mom) and her oldest daughter, Sis. The three girls were seated on one side of the table while Granny sat on the side nearest the kitchen, as a matter of convenience. Granny served herself only after serving everyone else, but before she could settle in her seat to begin to enjoy her meal, Grandpa Franklin's fist pounded on the table like a crude dinner bell, demanding more beer, more food, and more attention.

But it was washday. Granny had been up since 4 a.m.; Grandpa Franklin made it home for super around 7 p.m. Granny got up from her chair and went to the kitchen. The hickory wash stick stood leaning against the kitchen wall near the wood-burning stove. Granny entered the dining room with the beer as requested, but Grandpa Franklin was displeased with the speed of her service and continued to pound his fist on the table. "Woman, where's my goddamned beer?" he yelled as he voraciously shoveled the stew into his mouth, never looking up from his bowl.

But it was washday. Granny had been on her feet for 15 hours. Little Cora sat quietly as did everyone else, observing the scene that seemed for a while to play itself out in slow motion. Roberta, Little Cora, and Sis could all see Granny approach the table, holding the beer in one hand. Curiously though, she set the beer next to her own bowl.

Grandpa Franklin raised his fist one more time to pound the table, and—CRACK!!—It happened in a flash, sounding like a double-barreled shotgun firing. It was one of those scenes that must be replayed because even the most attentive observer undoubtedly missed a few frames. One moment, Grandpa Franklin was dominating the scene, yelling and pounding his fist on the table, and in the next, the six-feet-four-inch hunk of a coal miner was face down in his half-eaten bowl of hot stew. Behind him stood Granny holding the wash stick. She seated herself, placed the hickory stick on the floor, picked up the bottle of beer, and swallowed once. After a second swig she turned to Roberta, Little Cora, and Sis, saying, "Eat your stew."

Sis nervously stirred as if to stand in her ladylike fashion, but Granny flashed those blue-gray eyes at her firstborn and repeated, "I said, 'Eat … your … stew!'" With that, Sis quickly settled into her chair like her sister and niece. Their eyes turned to observe Grandpa, face down in his bowl. They wondered, *Is he breathing?* But no one dared check. In silence the three girls and Granny finished their supper, including dessert. The table was cleared as usual. Nothing was said. Grandpa Franklin was left blowing bubbles in his stew.

If there was any question about who was head of the Franklin household, it was forever settled. And it was settled on washday.

***

Prior to sixth grade, Little Cora remained oblivious to her racial heritage. Oskaloosa was insulated from racial diversity. The major exception was the Franklin family. Granny was biracial. Her husband was Dutch. Cora was the product of a Native

American mother and a biracial father.

Little Cora befriended the daughter of the superintendent of schools and their friendship blossomed for several years, which afforded a strained tolerance of her among the other schoolchildren. However, in 1929, a sixth grade class assignment would be the undoing of this friendship. The students were instructed to produce a family tree, and present it to the class. Granny worked with Little Cora to assure an accurate family tree, which Little Cora proudly presented to her classmates. Her mixed racial heritage was now out in the open. In an extraordinary measure taken by school administrators to separate her from her best friend, Little Cora was retained in sixth grade. This unfortunate and painful experience would leave an indelible and unsightly stain on the fabric of Cora Franklin's psyche. There was no academic reason to retain her. The experience was socially and psychologically devastating.

Cora remained in the Oskaloosa public schools for two more years, but in 1932 Granny sent her to live with her father in Chicago. Granny told her son that it was time for him to take responsibility for the child he abandoned so many years earlier.

This was a brilliant decision. Englewood High School opened in 1873 on Chicago's South Side. Cora's father was known as Mr. Frank in the Englewood community. The neighborhood was annexed by the city of Chicago in 1889 as part of a strategy to garner the World's Fair. Between the year of the annexation and 1920, Englewood's population grew by more than 86,000, largely the result of a steady stream of Irish, German, and Swedish immigrants. By the time Cora enrolled, the school's population was diverse. Cora blended in with her surroundings for the first time. Her complexion and mixed heritage were no longer an issue.

Cora clearly flourished in her father's care. She played violin in the youth symphony, sang in her high school chorus, and became a championship debater.

She also excelled in sports as a member of the girls' basketball team. Granny had planted the seeds of self-confidence in Cora back on the farm in Iowa. In Chicago those seeds took root and blossomed. It seemed that Cora finally had found a place for herself, drawing on her inner strength, and self-identifying as an extrovert. The experience of having been forced to repeat sixth grade was always there to challenge her self-esteem, and drive her tendency to overcompensate.

Granny chose to send Cora South to Wiley, a Historically Black College in east Texas, to complete her metamorphosis. This was another brilliant decision. Here Cora was among an economically diverse community of blacks who represented the entire color spectrum. No longer was Cora racially isolated. During her years at Wiley (1936 – 1942), Cora was exposed to a segment of the black diaspora supported by a strong and assertive community of mentors, academics, and politicians. When colorism raised its ugly head, Cora recalled the hardships she suffered because of her race while growing up in Iowa, and found solace in her ability to recognize and handle it. She did not know the love of her mother, the comfort of a nuclear family, or acceptance from her extended family. But Granny gifted her with self-confidence, a deep well from which she could drink freely whenever her wellbeing seemed parched by social discomfort or exclusion.

Over the course of her long life, Granny mastered many skills and amassed an infinite store of knowledge and wisdom. Living life fully for 101 years, with presence of mind and unobstructed mobility could not have come by chance alone, but with the impetus of her iron will, cunning, and tenacity. Having been born in the aftermath of the Civil War, Granny lived through: Reconstruction (1865 – 1877); the Jim Crow era (1877 – 1950's); World War I (1914 –1918); the ratification of the 19th amendment to the U.S. constitution in 1920; the Great Depression of the 1930's; World War II (1939 – 1945); the assassination of John F. Kennedy in 1963; and the signing of the Civil Rights Act of 1964, Executive Order 11246, issued by President Lyndon B. Johnson in 1965, which granted affirmative action to racial minorities and women for the first time in U.S. history.

In Granny's time, a common cold could be life threatening. She proved herself to be an expert in farming, mastering crop rotation, irrigation, and the purchase of livestock. She maintained her residence against harsh winters and flood waters. Therefore, it should come as no surprise that without a shred of formal training, she served as a skillful proctor to one of her sons as he worked to complete his Blackstone law studies in the late 1920's and early 1930's. That son went on to become a successful attorney in the Detroit Metropolitan area. Perhaps Granny knew as she studied law with her son that nothing in the universe is ever wasted.

From 1933 until 1942, Granny was left to run the farm alone, while her husband continued to work in the coal mines. Their eldest daughter, my Aunt Sis, was in Texas working as a housemother for the women's dormitory at Bishop College in Marshall. Granny enrolled her youngest daughter, my Aunt Bobbye in the same college. Granny' two sons were established in Chicago and in Detroit.

During the hard times of the Great Depression, as income from the farm all but dried up, Granny negotiated the sale of discrete plots of her farmland to generate much needed income, always insuring the preservation of her homestead. Granny also took in laundry from time to time, and provided cooking and handyman services to several elderly but financially independent neighbors.

A widow and former concert pianist rumored to be a relative of John Philip Sousa was one of Mahaska County's most renowned citizens. Granny provided meals and domestic services for this relative of the "The March King." Having performed in the concert halls of Europe, this dowager retired to one of many Quaker communities prevalent in the area. For nearly two decades, she was a major benefactor of Penn College, established in 1873 by a Quaker faction known as the Religious Society of Friends. While her relatives lived primarily along the eastern seaboard, the dowager chose the solace of a Quaker community in Iowa. In addition to providing domestic services and minor repairs around the house for which she was paid, Granny visited with the widow extensively. Eventually a genuine friendship developed between the two, as they became a familiar sight around the town. Having no affinity for her distant relatives, the dowager began to gift Granny with her personal possessions including China, crystal, and sterling flatware. Granny initially refused the gifts, but relented when the dowager expressed that she really had no desire to leave these items for "the vultures" (her estranged relatives) to pick through, over her grave.

Granny built a floor to ceiling china cabinet at one end of her dining room in which she attractively arranged these treasures. Knowing Aunt Bobbye's interest in pursuing a medical degree after graduating with honors from Penn College, the dowager purchased a new Model-A Ford, which provided Aunt Bobbye, Aunt Sis, and Mom transportation to and from Marshall.

Shortly after the widow died (around 1936), her heirs filed a lawsuit in Mahaska County, alleging Granny had stolen items from the "gullible and infirm benefactor of Penn College." As the trial date approached, Granny found herself unable to find a lawyer willing to represent her, and without a single witness to testify on her behalf. Having learned a great deal about the law as she proctored her son during his law courses, she had no choice but to represent herself.

Not wanting her ownership of the Model-A Ford to be placed in jeopardy, Granny prohibited her daughters and Mom from returning to Iowa until after the trial was over. During the jury trial, the prosecutor laid out his case with all the vitriol and disdain he could muster. When the prosecution rested, it was Granny's turn to address the court. It is important to understand that the jury pool would have consisted primarily of businessmen, most of whom were coal industry carpetbaggers. They had come to Mahaska County around the turn-of-the-century, whereas Granny had owned and occupied her land there since the late 1800's. She remembered when the judge and the prosecutor were born, and was at least 30 years older than anyone in the courtroom.

There being no witnesses to make her case, Granny stood in the well of the courtroom during her summation, and detailed her years of domestic service rendered to the deceased, absent any caregiving by relatives. She recalled the precise circumstances under which she reluctantly accepted the dowager's gifts. According to family lore, Granny addressed the prosecutors, the judge, the jury, and the general gallery with the facility ascribed to Clarence Darrow during the infamous Scopes Monkey Trial. The final words of her summation were ominous and foreboding. After alluding to the charges as false and unjust, she pointed to the judge, the prosecutor and the jury, saying, "I'll see all you sons of bitches dead and buried!" Clearly, they did not know what to make of her. First she wowed them with her intelligence and knowledge of the law. Then her dreadful pronouncement cloaked the courtroom in a stunned silence. Perceiving their astonishment, Granny walked gracefully and confidently from the courtroom.

Although Granny was found guilty of all charges, no Sherriff ever came to the Franklin farm to evict her or seize the items enumerated in the lawsuit. Within a year, however, both the judge and the prosecutor died of "natural causes." Granny saw the demise of all twelve jurors during the next decade. For many years, rumors persisted in Mahaska County that Granny had hexed her accusers. Folks were cautiously deferential to Mother Franklin, perhaps fearing that any disfavor from her may not end well for them.

Now, I never believed that Granny hexed anybody, but I am certain that she was an astute student of universal karma.

From Granny I learned compassion, assertiveness, and most importantly, the art of playing the hand you are dealt.

3 Mom

Our family had not been together for some years, so the Christmas of 1980 promised to be a special one. There was no great emphasis on Christmas gifts in our family and we never gave each other anything particularly personal. Still, the dilemma for my sister, Sandra, and me was what present to give our mother as a special expression of our love and respect for her. It was always difficult to buy presents for both our parents because they seemed to have everything.

As it happened, during Thanksgiving I visited Sedona, a small artists' community near Oak Creek Canyon and the Palatki Indian ruins, about an hour's drive from Phoenix, Arizona. While there, I chanced upon a handcrafted porcelain doll. She stood 26 inches tall and was dressed in white buckskin heavily adorned with colorful turquoise, coral, and white agate beads. On her feet were white buckskin moccasin-style boots, similarly beaded. A thick mane of silky black hair covered her head and framed her face. Her reddish tan complexion was exactly right. Seeing this exquisite work of art, I recalled immediately one of my mother's old and distant stories about never having owned a new doll. Although it was highly unusual for Sandra and me to collaborate on anything, I called her and suggested this doll could be the perfect solution to our dilemma. She agreed, and I made the purchase.

Three years earlier, Sandra had suffered an aneurism on Easter Sunday, and nearly died. She was hospitalized initially in Minneapolis where she worked, and then transported as soon as it was feasible to do so, to a hospital in Dallas where my parents lived. Sandra would be back in Dallas for the first time since spending four months in our parent's home, while Mom took care of her. Four months is long time, and I can imagine the two of them had enough of each other for a while. Around Thanksgiving that year, Sandra returned to Minneapolis to resume her life there. But this year, she would fly in from Minneapolis and I would drive up from Houston. The whole family would be together again. Everything just clicked.

Christmas Day finally arrived. My father's brother, Uncle Mac, and his wife were also present to celebrate with us. Dinner was exceptional. In my parents' home it was traditional to open presents on Christmas evening. At the appropriate time, Sandra and I together presented the doll to our mother. Although she accepted our gift graciously, she did not fuss over it. In fact, she did not seem particularly impressed with the doll. Still, I fell asleep that night feeling warm and gratified. Although the day could not compare to my childhood Christmases spent with Granny, it was quite memorable.

But in wee hours of the morning, I woke to what sounded like someone crying. Disoriented, I was unclear initially whether the weeping was part of an interrupted dream, some faded memory or, indeed, was actually real. It took me a few seconds to realize I was at my parent's home, in my old bedroom, and Sandra was asleep in the bedroom reserved for her. A Jack-and-Jill bathroom connected our two rooms.

I soon realized the weeping, though barely audible, was indeed real. Awake now, I decided to get up to investigate. In the dark, I bumped into my sister who had been awakened also, and apparently had the same idea. We gathered our senses and agreed to proceed quietly down the hallway in the direction of the muted sound beckoning us from the opposite side of the house. We made our way to the end of the hallway, turned and moved toward the living room. Strangely, the sound grew no louder, even as we drew closer to the perceived source. My sister led the way boldly, her bare feet stealthily traversing the marble tile floor in the entryway. The moonlight poured in through the floor-to-ceiling French windows at the front of the house, giving the interior a soft mournful glow, as the white brocade sofa positioned at an angle in the living room seemed to float on an ocean of ice blue carpeting. I joined my sister standing in the middle of the room where we found our mother sitting alone, crying. Her face was concealed by the darkness, but her soft and vague frame appeared forsaken and vulnerable. In her arms she held the porcelain doll. She caressed it, and cuddled it, and stroked its hair as if it were a newborn baby, and she were its mother.

Sandra and I sat on either side of our mother and held her tightly. After what seemed like hours she looked at each of us and said as she continued to cradle the doll, "This is the first time anyone gave me a doll of my very own. I always got the hand-me-downs, scratched and chipped, with worn clothing."

In that moment my sister and I became painfully aware that the doll awakened memories Mom had suppressed for over 60 years. In a way, our own sense of safety and security had been purchased by her pain and deprivation. Ironically, our gift, intended as a token of appreciation for our mother, became a gift of consciousness for my sister and me.

***

Cora Luella Franklin, the woman I knew as Mom, always displayed a strong and quiet persona. Cora grew to be a tall, statuesque young woman, sporting a figure that would become popularized by Jane Russell, a pinup girl, during World War II.

Self-improvement was her hallmark. Using her painful experience from sixth grade as a powerful motivator, she attained graduate degrees in education and library science in the 1960's.

My mother parlayed her Master's degrees into a position with the Upper Midwestern Regional School Board (UMRSB) whose purview included Iowa, Illinois, Michigan, Nebraska and Indiana. Mom attended planning sessions to investigate, evaluate, and document strategic initiatives designed to reinvent educational methodologies and infrastructures, while encouraging voluntary school desegregation. In addition to her work on the UMRSB, my mother was extremely instrumental in formulating the curriculum and administrative structures that defined the Bridgeway Project at Ulysses S. Grant Elementary in Waterloo:

> "... a school modeled on the Martin Luther King Jr. laboratory school in Evanston, Illinois, which attracted white students to a previously mostly black school by providing cutting-edge pedagogical innovations. The central idea behind the creation of such a school was that districts could persuade (rather than force) white parents to send their children to desegregated schools. Through a program of volunteer reverse busing, when Grant Elementary School reopened in the fall of 1970, it had a nearly perfect 50-50 balance of African-American and white children (Schumaker 2013, 353-385)."

When I was a high school senior, I vividly remember a tongue lashing I received as Mom picked me up from school to drive me to some extra-curricular event. After she asked, "How was your day?" I began to complain about what I believed to be the undeserved recognition of a classmate. Upon hearing my lament she challenged me by asking, "Who made you special that life should be fair to you?" For the next 20 minutes I was buried under a barrage of questions and perspectives, as she informed me that there would be a price to pay for everything worthwhile I dared to accomplish or possess. She emphasized that the price for me would be different each day, and it would never be exactly the same as Jimmy or Sally Anne down the street. She said, "You will have to decide whether you are willing to pay the price assigned to you, which could mean compromising some personal standard or ethic. If you should decide to pay your price by compromising a standard or ethic, don't complain. And if you should decide *not* to pay your price that day, don't complain."

I knew better than to interrupt her and stifled the responses that came to mind until she finished. My only desire was to hurry up and arrive at our destination so this lecture could end. When we finally arrived, she ended the lesson with a challenge before I could get out of the car. Turning to look directly into my eyes, she said, "Explain to me how you are hurt by having to know more." This turn in her monologue took me by surprise, and as I pondered her challenge, I quickly realized that life would afford me no easy pass. I would have to muster my knowledge, experience, and determination each time I sought to achieve a goal and claim a prize.

I always stood in awe of my mother's ability to construct extemporaneously a cogent, moral argument. The question ending her sermon would prompt me to rise to challenges yet to be presented without complaint. Through the years my application of the principles conveyed in this lecture would shield me from any feelings of entitlement, and reassure me I could attain anything I desired. I also learned to deemphasize the prize, but to focus on the quest. For in the journey lies the true treasure of an experience. Whether society cedes a trophy at the end of the journey is less important. It is sufficient to know I rose to the challenge, and proved myself *deserving* of the reward. The confirmation of success would be that all those who witnessed the effort would have intellectual certainty that recognition was in order, regardless of how the politics played out.

***

Like Granny, Miss Tread, and Dad, Mom had her own cadre of witticisms. She used to quip, "I may not start a fight in public, but I will damn sure end it in public!" If I was unclear about what she meant, all uncertainty would evaporate by the end of my senior year.

I began the year with the additional status as president of the student Senate, having been elected at the end of my junior year. I had visions of championing student rights, off-campus lunch privileges, improvements in school services, and producing one kick-ass senior prom. I actually started three weeks prior to the beginning of classes with my discovery of discretionary funding previously unknown to the student Senate. Due to my cunning (and to the administration's fear of my father's seat on the district school board), the funds were made available to me and my ad hoc committee without much protest. We chose one of the overflow study hall spaces on the first floor, which connected the new addition and the original school building. We converted the space to a student lounge and snack center, complete with modern café seating and new vending machines. I wanted this space to be inviting and uplifting for the students, a place where black and white students alike could mingle comfortably in an inviting, adult-like environment. As anticipated the students were stunned by the new student center, and my year was on a stellar trajectory.

My euphoria was tempered the day of our first student Senate meeting. We successfully covered all of the agenda items and staffed the action plan for the May senior prom. I believed we had comfortably sailed through the most challenging hurdles, and now our test would be simply to equal or surpass the success we had installing the student lounge. I intended to fully embrace my senior year. But at the conclusion of our first Senate meeting, a handful of students approached and questioned me about why I was treating a girl named Val so cruelly. I thought it was a prank, because I had never met Val, but the students merely scoffed and informed me that she was a member of the student Senate. My graduating class contained some 800 students, the high school population boasted nearly 2000 students, and there were roughly 40 student Senate members. I was intent on believing this was all part of some planned hazing of me due to my newly elected post. During the next few weeks, however, the interrogations persisted. Distinct factions in the school, including students, faculty, and administrators, all joined in. Okay – this was becoming a bit weird. I did not mention my conundrum to my parents, as I was certain once I found the anchor stitch, I could simply pull it and this ugly tapestry would unravel. How little I knew about social intrigue. Perhaps, *As the World Turns* or *General Hospital* could have prepared me for the world of deception and turbid gossip. I should have paid more attention. As it was, in no way was I prepared for the onslaught I would soon face.

Eventually a throng of students ambushed me between classes with the mysterious Val in tow. They were further angered when I displayed no visible recognition of the young lady. That was truly the first time I consciously laid eyes on her. I did not know that the assembled students were part of her posse. I did not know she had woven this *damsel in distress* fairytale into their deepest romantic fantasies. All the same, we had never met, we had never dated, I never "pinned" her, and I never dumped her. Although I must admit she was a bit homely to my taste and would have escaped my notice in any event, teachers and students alike believed her to be intellectually gifted. Therefore, the assumption was I would have been naturally attracted to her. Unbeknownst to me, my response to the ambush only affirmed her version of events. Just prior to Christmas vacation, I was summoned from class by the vice principal. This was not unusual. I was very active outside of the school in community endeavors for which I garnered several prestigious citizenship awards and scholarships. I was excused from class and went directly to the vice principal's office. When I arrived, he ushered me into his office and shut the door. So far, so good – everything seemed normal enough. I took a seat in front of his desk and inquired about his purpose in requesting the meeting, fully expecting him to brief me on some forthcoming event in the New Year. To my surprise, he turned to me and told me of his personal disappointment in my assault on this sweet young girl, Val. "What are you talking about?" I asked. But my denial only stoked his antagonism toward me. I was utterly confused. Although I knew him and he knew my father, neither I nor my father were close friends with this man. How could he possibly be offended by my behavior? After several minutes of inane conversation, I simply stood and told him he was nuts. With that I left his office and shut the door behind me.

During the Christmas holidays I confessed to my mother what had transpired the previous four months. I expressed my expectation that this would all resolve itself, to which she chuckled lightly. She listened intently, but silently, providing no hint of her thoughts. She simply cast that reassuring gaze my way, and told me it would be alright. At the conclusion of the Christmas break I returned to school and found the behavior of my fellow students and teachers to be unchanged, with the exception that the focus now shifted to inquiries concerning the identity of the person I was planning to take to the prom. Tickets for the prom would go on sale the first week of March, and preparations would be finalized in January and February. My response was that I wasn't planning to attend the prom, which prompted a myriad of reactions – surprise, bewilderment, suspicion, and disgust – among my detractors. I managed to get through the first few weeks of ticket sales, but the inquiries about my prom date persisted. I reverted to my defense mechanism of choice, deciding to simply ignore people with that air of dismissal for which I was well known.

The first Saturday in April my mother informed me we had an errand to run and to be ready to leave the house around 10:00 a.m. I dressed well and met her at the car. She drove me across town to the home of Mrs. Wright who was expecting us. Standing beside her was her daughter, Charmaine. She and I had been enrolled in my mother's class in sixth grade at Grant Elementary. I had not seen her since junior high. A new high school opened our sophomore year, and we ended up attending different schools. Charmaine had blossomed into quite the poised and voluptuous young woman. We were invited into Mrs. Wright's dining room where we were served drinks and cake, as she and my mom continued a discussion that apparently had been underway for several months. Charmaine and I sat quietly listening, but not speaking. Then my Mom turned to me and said definitively that I was taking Charmaine to the senior prom. Her declaration was sanctioned by a nod from Mrs. Wright. With that, the table was cleared and we all got in my mom's car.

Mom drove to her favorite boutique, a place familiar to me, as I had often accompanied her to private showings the owners arranged upon their return from buying trips in Chicago and New York. But today it was Charmaine, not Mom, who was there for a final fitting. Mrs. Wright and my mother had chosen an exquisite off-the-shoulder white and ivory silk brocade evening gown tailored to Charmaine's figure with such precision it looked as if it had been spray-painted on, yet it was not uncomfortably tight. The gown was split in the back up to the knee. The boutique owners fitted Charmaine with matching 3-inch heels. This was a grownup ensemble. Charmaine looked stunning in that gown, and to my surprise moved elegantly and gracefully about the room in those 3-inch pumps. I shook my head and laughed silently.

The following week, as I was again bombarded with questions about my prom date, I shocked everyone when I casually mentioned that I was taking Charmaine Wright. No one knew who Charmaine was – at least no one within Val's posse. One of my elementary school classmates, Fred Allen, walked me to class and asked if Charmaine was the Charmaine we knew in elementary school. I told him she was, but that he would not recognize her today. Fred had always quietly had my back. He was captain of our championship football team, and although we did not hang out together, he remained my steadfast advocate. Prior to my announcement, Val had played the role of the abandoned damsel who did not know how she was going to endure attending the prom unescorted. Miraculously, within days of my announcement, she had a date. I was beginning to catch on to the depths of this choreographed drama of deceit. Val aimed to force me into capitulating for my alleged ill-treatment of her, and to publicly ask for her forgiveness. From this I suppose she believed she would achieve some kind of elevated status, having manipulated the son of Dr. Harvey. It was sick and twisted, but it was Waterloo, after all – a Midwestern *Peyton Place* sans Ryan O'Neal, Mia Farrow, and Dorothy Malone. Still, the drama was salacious enough in a rustic, farm-belt kind o' way.

A few weeks later Val arranged for me to meet with her in the orchestra rehearsal room. When I arrived she turned to me with tears in her eyes, and apologized for the plot she launched against me. I believed that her tears were genuine, but I would not forgive her for the anxiety and embarrassment she caused me or for the deception she visited upon other unwitting students. I told her I wished never to speak with her again, as I left her sobbing in the rehearsal room.

The East High senior prom was a commercial success. It was a sold-out affair. I was unaware how extensively the Val-Reginald saga had saturated the Waterloo community. I reserved a table, but it was our entrance that was the sweetest revenge. Charmaine was stunning! All of the girls were wearing their pastel puffy sleeved Junior Petite dresses, as Charmaine walked in like Hallie Berry, Vivica Fox, and Naomi Campbell all rolled into one. As we approached our table, she glided across that room slowly, holding her pearl beaded clutch casually in one hand, and resting her free arm upon mine. Some of the students from my elementary school recognized her, but to most in the room she was a stranger. Charmaine was courteous, kind, and endearing. Everyone wanted to talk to her, and all were shocked that she was from Waterloo Central High school. People wanted to know how we got together. Charmaine kept our secret, selling the act effortlessly because it was rooted in genuine joy and excitement. After all, she was rewarded with a very expensive evening gown, and was wearing a string of her mother's pearls. Her hair had been exquisitely coiffed in a tight French role and her beautiful silky black locks fell freely into her face. She sat properly as would any seasoned lady, as she wore that gown till it cried, "I'm not bad, I'm just drawn that way."

Mom damn sure knew how to end a fight in public!

***

I was always proud of my mother—her stature, her wit and her confidence. She used to say, "When you enter a room, own it. That way no one would dare question your right to be there."

Nonetheless, my mother's gregarious personality was a challenge for me at times. During my first semester at the University of Iowa, I did not own a car and relied on my parents to pick me up for weekend visits home. I did not have a problem with this arrangement and actually looked forward to those trips. The first time my mother came to pick me up, she was late. Or at least I thought she was. This was 1973, and there were no cell phones. A commitment to rendezvous had to be made in advance and kept. My mother was characteristically punctual, so her tardiness raised my concern that she may have suffered some inconvenience, perhaps even an accident. My first thought was to call my father to confirm when Mom left home, but I thought better of this, not wanting to raise undue worry. Each floor of my 13-story coed dormitory had a reception/conference area located at the end of the hallway overlooking a small parking lot. I decided to make intermittent trips to the reception area on my floor to see if I could locate her car in the parking lot and therefore confirm her arrival.

Earlier that year my mother purchased a new Buick Riviera, which was a combination muscle car and luxury coupe. She paid $7,500 in cash for the car, which was loaded with every customized option available. My father was vocal about his distaste for the amount of money she spent. This argument was the first I ever witnessed between my parents. Mom reminded Dad that she used her own money to buy the car, and if he didn't like it, he need never put his ass in it. Case closed – permanently.

Upon my first trip to the reception area, I scanned the parking lot and immediately spotted the distinctive profile of the boat-tailed Buick, sporting rich sky-blue metallic paint, a white landau roof and two thin white pinstripes. It looked like a speeding bullet, even when parked. Seeing the car I knew she had arrived, so I took the elevator down to the first floor lobby. It was almost 6 o'clock on a Friday evening. Most students had already left campus for the weekend, so the lobby should have been empty. I exited the elevator walking swiftly towards the door with the intention of going to the parking lot where I assumed Mom would be waiting.

I made it only halfway across the lobby before I noticed about 30 students gathered to one side engaged apparently in a conversation as they sat cross legged in a circle on the floor. The familiar sound of my mother's voice, recounting some bizarre story to those assembled stopped me in my tracks. I was mortified. I turned to see that these students who should be out seeking libations and listening to the latest rock music were sitting entranced, their eyes fixed on my mother. Suddenly Mom said to the crowd, "Oh, there's my baby!" In an instant I went from shock to embarrassment as I tried frantically to make my feet move backwards and provide my escape to the elevator. But my mother's eyes and broad smile found me standing motionless. The crowd of students turned and looked at me, almost cheering, which only added to my embarrassment. I thought, "I have to live with these people. How could you do this to me?" Habit forced me to walk toward my mother as if tethered to a fishing line as she reeled me in. She stood, hugged me and offered more words of introduction to this gaggle of students. That episode established me as somewhat of a celebrity in the dorm. In the days and weeks that followed, students whom I did not know greeted me enthusiastically by name.

Over the next 18 months the unwanted attention morphed into a bizarre following of students who would insist on traveling home with me to spend the weekend with my parents. I never got to go *away* on spring break or holidays. I would make plans, but my schoolmates would invariably ask, "When are we leaving for your parents' house?" I would end up with four or five students following me home. I always warned them that my mom was crazy and likely to say or do anything. But that did nothing to dissuade her fan club. Decades later I was forced to admit that there was something about my parents that the other kids found magical. It took years to understand how fortunate I was to have grown up around these people. Apparently, my uniquely rich relationship with my parents was something my contemporaries did not have in their lives, but fortunately, they found a way to fill this void by adopting my parents, especially my convivial mother.

***

In my early twenties, I came to know my mother's mischievous side. As I established my career in Houston's petrochemical industry, Mom visited each year during her spring break. One evening while we were stuck in rush-hour traffic returning to my house from an outing, Mom interrupted the sound of the idling car engine to share memories of her college days. She began, "When I was in college, it wasn't enough to have the right dress for the right shoes and the right makeup, to be ready for a party. Yes, in those days it was important to make your entrance. But a girl wasn't ready for a party unless she had confirmed at least three dates." I knew not to inject myself into one of her monologues, as it was impossible to know which rabbit hole would swallow me up. So after an uncomfortable silence, she continued, "I guess you want to know the purpose of the three dates." Truthfully, I did not want any such details, but she took my nonresponse as consent and continued. "Well, a lady has to have the proper escort when she enters an event. But usually the proper escort (guy number one) is boring. Proper, but boring. So it's best to have preplanned a rendezvous with a hunk (guy number two), who would already be at the party to keep things spicy. I suppose you may be wondering about the reasoning behind guy number three? …This is the boy who likes you more than you like him. In case guy number one is offended when learning of guy number two, a girl needs a guaranteed way home. That's the purpose for guy number three. He will happily see you home safely, as this is an opportunity for him to be with you."

I sat speechless for a moment. I couldn't decide whether my mom had been outrageously clever or simply a slut. Later that evening I called Sandra in Minneapolis and told her, "You should have been kinder to Mom because she had a foolproof plan for how to manage men. She knew how to do what you were only *trying* to do. Compared to her you were Amateur Night!"

Yes, Mom remained an enigma. She was funny, mischievous, fearless, loving, tenacious and engaging. She had the cunning to disarm her adversaries and win the favor of those who were uncertain about her place in the social pecking order. Her razor-sharp wit and keen powers of observation rendered her a force of nature. She was my best friend and my anchor.

She taught me how to fight my battles without resorting to pejorative epithets or physical violence. My relationships with my mother, godmother and Granny virtually assured that I would never be intimidated by strong-willed women or my elders or any adversity whatsoever. I would summon this strength time and time again in my battle for survival.

I love you, Mom… and I miss you!

4 Miss Tread

I lived in Waterloo until my sophomore year in college. In the fifties and sixties, front doors in Waterloo were routinely left unlocked, except when the occupants went on vacation. But few people ever took a vacation. Why travel? This was Waterloo. What else was there to see? Everything conceivable could be found within a 3.5-mile radius. There were 36 bowling alleys, three roller-skating rinks, and three movie theatres, including a drive-in with a gigantic screen where patrons could count on seeing the latest blockbuster movie.

With 75,000 residents, Waterloo was home to one of the largest populations between Des Moines, the capital, and a far off and alien metropolis called Chicago. Then, as now, the economy was dominated by the agricultural and food processing industries. Several hundred family farms dotted the landscape of Black Hawk and surrounding counties. The large, pristine farms on the outskirts of the city with straight furrows of corn, soybeans, oats, and wheat were a testament to the largely Germanic heritage of many residents.

Fresh produce, processed meat, and livestock rolled down the tracks to places unknown courtesy of the Illinois Central Railroad, which employed nearly 30,000 people, together with John Deere Tractor Works and Rath Packing Company. About 10,000 Waterloo residents were black, having arrived from the share cropping fields of Mississippi as strike breakers for the Illinois Central Railroad in the early 1900's. Jobs were plentiful. There was no war. Life was predictable. People were content (or at least they were complacent).

The Cedar River divided the town. The East Side (actually located north of the river) was home to blue collar workers, while merchants and professionals lived on the West Side (south of the river). But East Side or West Side, the slaughterhouse was an equal opportunity polluter.

There were no cell phones back then. "Friends" were not some distant electronic entity, but real people—neighbors, church members, and co-workers—who greeted each other, argued over minor issues, and discussed the events of the day face to face. Dogs ran freely in the neighborhood, but this was not a nuisance since everyone knew each dog's name and owner. A whistle or a name called was enough to get a wandering dog's attention, and ordering the animal to go home would have precisely the desired effect.

Children walked to school with their lunch pails and skipped across parks under the watchful eyes of neighbors relaxing on the front porch or weeding their flower beds. Kidnapping was unheard of and there were no rumors, confirmed or otherwise, of child abuse.

Life was perfect. I had Mom and Dad and we all had Effie Lincoln Treadwell.

There is a concept in most cultures that approximates what we call "guardian angels", a physical or supernatural presence whose purpose is to guide and protect us. Believers of the supernatural presence assert that there is a connection between this physical dimension and some parallel or coexisting plane where a consciousness external to us interacts with our senses. Such encounters may manifest as a waking dream, apparition, angel, or a vision of some deceased relative or mentor. The impact of these encounters is commonly described as a kind of heightened awareness or clarity of perception, resolving struggles of consciousness between right and wrong, good and evil, or precipitating in some manifest adjustment of intention or commitment or will. According to one school of thought, each of us comes into this world with a higher purpose and our guardian angels appear from time-to-time or indeed walk among us perennially to provide gentle guidance or strength to achieve this purpose.

I have no problem believing all this. My early life was profoundly impacted by the physical and perennial presence of the woman I knew as Miss Tread, my godmother. She was surely my guardian angel. Actually, she was my family's guardian angel.

Miss Tread was born in New Orleans' French Quarter in the 1880's. She moved to Waterloo at the dawn of the Great War, establishing a boarding house there. She was a descendent of some combination of African enslaved persons and South American Indians brought to Louisiana by European settlers in the mid-1600's. A more precise heritage is impossible to know, but the stories she shared of her life as a little girl on the streets of New Orleans portrayed a child whose very survival depended on her ability to successfully integrate a variety of cultures and religious systems. She was familiar with African spirituality and African-based cultures from Haiti, West Africa, Cuba, and the Dominican Republic. At the same time, she attended Catholic school and was familiar with the European interpretation of Christianity. Interestingly, there is a dynamic interaction between Voodoo cultures and Christianity that I will not explore here, but clearly Miss Tread learned very early in her life to resolve or negotiate any inconsistencies among the belief systems and rituals endemic to this rich mix of cultures. She used to talk about being able to see spirits when she was a young girl. Her own mother talked with certainty of the existence of another dimension, but cautioned her daughter on being too curious about it.

Not surprisingly, Miss Tread was a deeply spiritual woman with the ability to understand the nexus between human conflict and the "demons" of addictive behavior, sexual promiscuity, social manipulation, power, and greed. She met those under the spell of such influences not only with a sense of grace, charity, and empathy, but also with a strong resolve to prevent these individuals from causing undue harm to the innocent or gullible. Those who may have harbored ill intentions could be disarmed by her sharp wit and infectious smile. I never believed she was on a mission to save the world, but in addition to her role as my guardian, she was a caretaker and esteemed elder within the greater community. She enjoyed respect far and wide.

For a time, Miss Tread owned and operated a thriving boardinghouse, providing a safe haven to a wealth of African Americans who could not find lodging in motels or hotels serving whites. From World War I through the early days of World War II, Miss Tread played host to the likes of Count Basie, Duke Ellington, the Neville Brothers, the Mills Brothers, and B. B. King as they traveled the circuit, usually by car (as this was safer) from south of the Mason Dixon Line to the show palaces of Chicago, and on to New York. Emerging politicians, graduate students, and entrepreneurs were also counted among her patrons. Her boardinghouse was a welcome respite for those travelling back and forth as well as those desperate to escape permanently the Jim Crow South, seeking a chance to fulfill their dreams. I never knew the moniker of the boardinghouse, but I have intellectual certainty that Miss Tread became famous in the region for bringing her other-worldly Creole flavors and textures from the "old country" of New Orleans to this farming community in the Midwest.

Effie Lincoln met her husband, Ben Treadwell, in Waterloo shortly after World War I. He was among those strike breakers brought to town from Mississippi. A quiet man, Mr. Tread, as we called him, was a master diesel mechanic early on. He stood six feet four inches, was fair-skinned with broad chiseled facial features, and sported a physique that could rival any bodybuilder. He shaved with a straightedge razor, and could have been a model for one of Michelangelo's statues. Hard labor and the various jobs he survived as a young man growing up in the South were responsible for his strong and trim physique. A veteran of World War I, Mr. Tread remained a faithful husband to his wife until her death in the late 1970's.

In 1936 Miss Tread closed her boardinghouse and built a home in Waterloo. The bungalow boasted the latest architectural features, upscale appointments, and (until the 1950's) the only telephone in the neighborhood. She and her husband transformed the vacant acre of land adjacent to their home into a rich and vibrant garden, one quarter of which was corn, while root vegetables, strawberries, and pear, apple, and cherry trees were also part of the mix. A grape arbor defined three sides of the garden and peonies bloomed along the remaining edge. My godmother was in heaven walking barefoot in the garden, blessing each plant with her individual attention. As an excellent cook with an extensive regional reputation, Miss Tread never opened a restaurant, but continued to use her culinary skills to welcome newcomers and ease the burdens of those experiencing personal tragedies and other disruptive events. It was a singular honor for a family to receive a meal prepared by her.

When my parents relocated from Iowa City to Waterloo in 1955, following my father's graduation from the University of Iowa College of Dentistry, it was inevitable they would meet this amazing woman. It is not important *how* they met, but critically important that their paths did indeed cross, for Miss Tread would have a deeply profound and enduring impact on my family and me.

In truth, both Miss Tread and my parents were somewhat out of place in Waterloo. She became a welcome counselor and sage to my parents. She was the only person I knew who could call my Dad aside for a private conference. From time to time, Miss Tread would dismiss my mother, my sister, and me through artfully executed cues. "Doc," she would say with a twinkle in her eye, "have some coffee." And we all knew to vacate the premises, while Dad received private counsel from this wise old woman. We never knew what they discussed, but Dad would come home several hours later and for months his spirit would seem brighter and his steps lighter. It was as if she provided a pressure valve, which allowed him to endure life among the farmers and laborers of Waterloo. I suspect my parents' 54-year marriage could be attributed in no small measure to Miss Tread.

To my great advantage, Miss Tread was practically the only caretaker I knew, aside from my parents. Her plump and sturdy frame measured a mere five feet. She was brown-skinned with sweet round cherubic features and small hands with manicured nails, always sans nail polish, but sporting gorgeous art deco style wedding rings. She loved White Shoulders powder, lotion, and perfume. Although plagued with psoriasis on her legs, which bled at times, she soaked them in Epsom salt, wrapped them up and never complained. As she was meticulous about her personal appearance, she wore support hose to mask her skin condition. At home, aprons with a flower or fruit motif were a permanent fixture around her waist. Her shoulder-length dark hair, graying around the temples, was often pulled back in a bun. Her head was characteristically unadorned except with a hat on Sundays. She seemed to be always washing her hands and cleaning her nails owing to the time she spent in the kitchen. She watched Jimmy Swaggart on television (until he was defrocked), and held the Supremes, Ed Sullivan, and Chet Huntley in equal esteem. She read her Bible faithfully, but never proselytized, preferring instead to live her faith. My dad made her a set of dentures, which she wore only occasionally, apparently feeling more comfortable without them. Mr. Tread was powerful in physique, but Miss Tread *was* the power. Her small sparking eyes could hold you transfixed in their gaze.

Prior to kindergarten, I spent my days in her company. Our classroom was her kitchen and dining room, a magical place to be. She taught me to read and write at the age of three. Sitting at her dining room table as she consumed her morning chicory coffee and saltine crackers, we "discussed" the news of the day. Although the emphasis was on local goings on, she also filled me in on regional and even national news, speaking to me as if I were another adult. She shared rich and captivating stories and parables that prompted me to ask questions and explore concepts of morality and ethics. I learned the skill of asking questions and came to an understanding of ideas far exceeding my years. This skill was reinforced by my parents throughout my life.

Our conversations were so rich and exciting to me that I could recall and review them with improved understanding as I grew older. As a young adult, I learned how very unique this aspect of my childhood was. In college I would see my peers struggling with crisis management under circumstances whose resolution seemed very clear to me with respect to both the perceived options and consequences. Neither my godparents nor my parents hid much from me. They were always present and available to fill in the gaps and provide me with a strong sense of security so that it was safe to discuss and explore any issues or concepts that my young mind could raise.

Since my grandparents were unknown to me, Miss Tread became a surrogate grandmother. If life became dreary or heavy from time to time, Miss Tread provided a respite for us all. She was my Muse, as reliable as the rising sun, shining the light of her wisdom freely on my life.

I imagine I was a somewhat precocious and challenging child, with my fair share of quirks. For one thing, I never developed the love of peanut butter and jelly shared my most children. Not for lack of trying. The chemistry of my saliva, however, could not break down the darned stuff. No matter the medium—bread, crackers, celery, or other conveyance—the peanut butter would dissolve leaving a gummy glob of inert matter in my mouth. Although I really liked the texture, crunch and taste of all kinds of nuts, peanut butter was a "food group" that I could not conquer.

Understanding this, Miss Tread took care to prepare glorious sweet cream butter and jelly sandwiches especially for me. The thing that made these treats particularly delicious is that she made her own jams, jellies, and fruit butters. Like many women in the community, she was an expert canner, sparing us the ills of chemical preservatives.

The food preparation for the canning process itself was accomplished with great care and planning, which included carefully peeling the fruit or vegetable. Sometimes blanching or slight dehydration was part of the process. Watchful eyes monitored the moisture content of the produce to be preserved. Canned items had a shelf life ranging from one to five years.

Nearly every house in Iowa was built with a root cellar, densely packed earth framed with semi-porous cinderblocks providing natural refrigeration throughout the year. Those canned fruits would be retrieved from time to time from the root cellar and further processed into the fantastic jellies and fruit butters used to fashion my sandwiches. Even as a small child I was involved in harvesting, washing, and monitoring the plants as they dried. Although too small to actively assist in the cooking phases of preservation, I was eager to observe the process from beginning to end. The importance of this or that procedure was carefully explained to me, but I needed little encouragement as I benefitted directly from the final product.

But we were not vegetarians. A few live fowls were placed in the root cellar several days before Mr. Tread slaughtered them. Processing the birds involved placing the feathered carcasses in her huge farmhouse sink and pouring boiling water carefully over them. Humming hymns in a slow meter as she worked, Miss Tread used a pair of pliers and wire cutters to painstakingly pluck the feathers from the birds. This was followed by a bath of saltwater into which she placed the plucked carcasses and then with great care scraped the skin with a wire brush to remove any fragment of feathers still anchored in the skin. Equal portions of strength and skill were necessary to avoid tearing the skin. Repeated baths cleaned the carcasses inside and out and tenderized the meat, a bonus for slow cooking. Miss Tread seasoned the birds and cooked them until the meat fell off the bone, but was never dry or overcooked. Again, the secret was patience and careful monitoring.

The incredibly delicious meals Miss Tread prepared as part of her community outreach, not only contained fruits and vegetables from her enormous garden, but also chicken and turkey, prepared as described. I assisted in packing those glorious dinners and accompanying Mr. Tread to make deliveries.

Such was my playtime.

Raised by her grandmother on a farm, my own mother was no stranger to these cooking techniques. Miss Tread seemed to appreciate my mother's cooking skills. They bridged the generations separating them by sharing their mutual appreciation for the art of cooking.

I remember one occasion when Miss Tread called Mom with an "urgent" problem. She intimated that the issue had something to do with her grape jelly, but she was unwilling to discuss the details on the phone. This was serious. Mom rushed down with me in tow. Once in the kitchen, Miss Tread went through each painstaking step in her recipe for making grape jelly only to reach the point at which she could not get the substance in the pot to jell. This was a longstanding mystery she hoped Mom could help her solve. Mom reached into her pocket and pulled out a packet of Sure-Jell…and voila! Mystery solved. Miss Tread was astonished. It was magic!

She made Mom swear never to reveal her use of this newfangled product. Mom agreed to provide her with a steady supply so that Miss Tread never had to risk getting caught buying the stuff at the grocery store. Mom and I laughed about this story for years.

I have wondered often the conundrum I would have suffered had I been placed in the care of a 12-year-old.

Miss Tread and her friends were 60-plus years my senior. Their stories were rich with color, angst, and triumph. Many of these women were survivors of spouses who died in World War I or II. In particular, I remember a gracious lady by the name Lyda Paige. Mother Paige was at least 20 years older than my godmother. Doing the math I guess she may have been about 10 years older than Granny. I remember her as the esteemed elder in our Methodist church. I was awestruck by the notion that there were people even older than my godmother to whom she looked for guidance and encouragement. Observing these near-centenarians, I became comfortable with the idea that the treasure of knowledge and wisdom was rooted in long-lived experience and personal triumph. But to be honest, Mother Page made the best damned hot chocolate on the planet.

My "playmates" had money and cars, and provided me with an unwavering sense of security. I felt free to explore the world without fear. In that sense I enjoyed a charmed childhood filled with wonder and ever expanding knowledge. I did not know dismissal, isolation, hunger, or abandonment. I was not always the center of attention, but as a member of my family I was respected and not marginalized by my age and inexperience. This instilled in me a sense of worth, self-respect, and confidence. I was nurtured to rely on a special kind of courage and character.

How could I have been afforded these benefits under the tutelage of a 12-year-old?

***

"Toots" is a slang term of endearment, usually meaning "my dear," or "babe", but can also be used pejoratively (for example, "dumb ass"). I never heard anyone except my godmother use this term. When it crossed her lips, I understood her meaning, which was emphasized with the inflection, tone or sharpness of delivery. When my godmother pressed a point with me, almost invariably, "Toots" was my alert to pay close attention. Sure to follow was some particular wisdom or insight or inspiration to empathize with another's pain or disappointment, or to suggest an urgency or sincerity of goodwill.

"Toots," she would say, "always be true to yourself. Never pretend to be someone you are not. Should you turn a corner and find yourself in an unfamiliar neighborhood, hold fast to your roots. The inhabitants know you are a stranger, but will respect your individuality, and help you to return to where you belong. Should you attempt to fake membership in that strange community, they will eat you alive."

"If a man has dirt under his fingernails and he is not either a mechanic or a farmer, be wary. That man is untrustworthy, and his true purpose will be revealed in time."

"A leopard is born with a finite number of spots. One may try to hide spots or add spots or substitute stripes for spots, but in the end the leopard has the same number of spots at its death that it had at birth."

"Everyone climbs Fools Hill, especially when young. But when your old, tired ass is still climbing Fools Hill, it's an ugly site!"

"Climb down off the cross. Somebody else needs the wood."

"If you think you have power, try ordering somebody else's dog to do tricks."

My godmother did not mouth vacuous platitudes to hear herself talk or to bolster her importance. She lived these axioms daily. They conveyed her sense of social justice, her love of community, and her active community service. They were freely shared in the hopes of sparing others the consequences of naivety, self-absorption, and other human frailties. As a child I could not appreciate these sayings, but Miss Tread's inimitable delivery seared them into my consciousness.

Whenever there was a worthy community project, a health crisis or a tragedy in need of her support, I observed Miss Tread as she jumped into "action" sitting in her recliner, telephone in her lap, calling people around the country, asking for their financial support. Her tagline was, "Toots, we could really use your help," and magically pledges flowed in totaling twenty, thirty or forty thousand dollars—and this was in the early 1960's. It took years for me to piece together the jigsaw puzzle of her fundraising prowess, because she had no glossy marketing brochures or flashy commercials. She simply asked people for their support.

Over time, the pieces to the puzzle fell into place, revealing an incredibly stunning picture of skill, altruism, and goodwill. For starters, she never called anyone haphazardly or too often. And she only called people she knew or whom she had helped at some time in their life. Her pleas for assistance were received with open arms, often as an opportunity for those she had once assisted to pay it forward. Her contacts no doubt included some of the famous people who patronized her boarding house years earlier. She never, never compromised a confidence or sought personal recognition or glory. Funds flowed from around the country through her and out into the community. She was the quintessential fundraising "clearinghouse."

A huge piece to this puzzle was a long-standing collaboration Miss Tread nurtured with a woman I will refer to as Lizzie, who was probably Creole. Lizzie was another peculiar figure in this farming and factory community. She was beautiful and exotic.

Lizzie did not visit often, but several times a year she would arrive at Miss Tread's house in a grand 1950's Cadillac that sparkled like a brand-new silver dollar. It was a pastel green like the color of young grass, and encased in chrome. A chariot on whitewall tires. It was a convertible, even though no one else in Waterloo had a convertible. She wore high heels and expensive perfume. She was always exquisitely dressed and gloved, which I found odd since her visits fell in the middle of the week. Freshly baked tea cakes, angel food cake, and other delicacies I could not pronounce, signaled these meetings. There would be a fresh pot of chicory coffee brewing during lunch to allow it enough time to steep. Lizzie would arrive just after my lunch and before my afternoon nap, and never failed to have a little treat in her purse for me, which I accepted with a nod from Miss Tread. Afterwards, I was dispatched to play outside in my godmother's back yard and garden, a place that would have inspired J.R. Tolkien's Shire. I was happy to go, for I knew that my nap would be reprieved, and I would get to sample the special pastries after Lizzy departed, perhaps I would even get a sip or two of that chicory coffee with heavy cream and sugar. Yum!

Three outstanding truisms condense the lessons indelibly woven into the fabric of my character by my godmother: never apologize for who you are; preserve the integrity of your character and that of those around you; and refuse to partake in groupthink. Her elaborate food preparation rituals taught me that great reward may be reaped through patience and careful planning, and quelled any tendencies toward instant gratification. Whenever I encounter a predicament that conjures one of her sayings, I smile as I glean an ever fuller understanding of her wisdom.

As for Lizzie, the events of a certain Easter Sunday a few years later would shed light on this mysterious woman and her friendship with my godmother.

5 Lizzie

It was Easter Sunday 1963, and all the Methodists in our perfect little community—and perhaps a few Baptists—were worshipping in our new church building.

The 11 o'clock service at Payne Memorial African Methodist Episcopal Church had long since crept past the halfway mark. The choir had moved the congregation to an emotional highpoint, and the sermon was delivered with brilliance and power. Many, many prayers had been lifted up, beseeching the Almighty, and the contents of the collection plates were safely on their way to Church coffers.

The men of the Trustee Board sat in the front row on one side of the center aisle, while the Stewardesses, sat on the other side, dressed in their usual white uniforms. These women nurtured and protected the moral fiber and prestige of the church. They had the power of censorship. It was not a good idea to offend a

Stewardess. Miss Tread, my playmate, guardian angel, and godmother, was not a Stewardess. She stood apart, exceeding in a way the standing of any individual Stewardess. As the "mother" of the church her status was unparalleled, and her wisdom was unquestioned.

Sunrise Service went off without a hitch, thanks to a group of mostly women taking up several pews directly behind the trustees. They were the committed congregants who attended the 6 a.m. Sunrise Service, ushering, helping to serve breakfast, or contributing in some other essential way to early morning events— and then stayed for 11 o'clock Service. There was no shortage of those willing to make this sacrifice. On the contrary, there was competition to be counted in their ranks. There were three reasons for this. The first was to impress others with their piety. The second was recognition. They were given a "VIP pass" including priority seating directly behind the Trustees, and the Pastor himself extolled their commitment from the lectern. The third and perhaps most important reason was the 11 o'clock service was the Main Event. It was a chance to strut and fret their hour upon the Payne Memorial stage.

I sat next to Miss Tread, who sat where she *always* sat: in the second row, behind the Stewardess in the seat next to the center aisle. Even in her absence, no one else dared sit there. Today, Miss Tread was dressed in her new "burial suit"—one in a long line of tailor-made suits purchased each year, just in case she should transition to glory. If she was not dead by Easter, she unpacked the outfit carefully and wore it, then religiously ordered another masterpiece for the following year. This one was a powder blue fitted dress of textured silk with a matching coat that perfectly aligned with the hem of the dress. She also wore new shoes covered in the same wonderful powder blue fabric. Did I mention her hat? It was truly a work of art. She was properly dusted with lilac powder and there was a hint of White Shoulders perfume on the lace handkerchief holding the treasure: marvelous white candies with the chewy spearmint jelly centers. It was my job to wrest stealthily the candy, piece by piece, from its hiding place in the lace handkerchief. This was the game we played.

Miss Tread suffered from "sugar" diabetes and gout, particularly in her legs, which swelled painfully. Due to her condition, she took to attending church services only on first Sundays, when communion was served. She soaked and salved her legs all week so that they would cooperate with her support hose on Sunday.

I was very close to extracting the last luscious piece of candy from Miss Tread's handkerchief. After church my family would dine at her table. The candy was the only thing that could keep my mind off the feast waiting at her house. Although I was eager for services to end, everything was taking longer than usual because the new church overflowed with people. There were people seated in the Narthex, as the balcony was full. Many had overflowed onto the portico capping the Narthex, and the kids (usually dispatched to the balcony) were in the basement still seated quietly, listening to the goings on above. *Hurry, hurry. I am nearly out of candy and dinner is waiting. Let's serve the tasteless wafers and the Welch's Grape Juice, have the benediction and get home to dinner!* Such were the workings of my eight-year-old mind.

In my position beside the queen, the mother of the church, I got to see and hear everything. And what a sight it was. Every woman tried to outdo the other. The congregation was a sea of marvelous textures and pastel colors. As music played, nodding hats, each one bigger and more ornate than the next, rocked like sail boats moored in a marina. Gloved hands held lace handkerchiefs, and there was so much support restraining those ample female frames that Platex surely scored record annual profits that year. The music flowed like a soft curtain in a breeze, as everyone lined up single file down the center aisle for altar call, that solemn procession ending at the altar railing where each kneeled and prayed. This was each woman's chance to sachet around and show off her trussed up figure in her new outfit complete with coordinating handbag and shoes. Nothing more grand had been staged since Judy Garland and Fred Astaire strolled down turn-of-the-century Park Avenue in Vincent Minelli's *Easter Parade*.

All paid respect to Miss Tread as they quietly and regally rose from the altar and returned to their pew. But a stranger who stood out from the rest, also nodded at Miss Tread, who smiled broadly and nodded approval in return. But wait – I knew this woman. It was Lizzie. I was surprised because I had never seen her at church before.

In the background the Bishop with outstretched arms was enjoining the Holy Spirit to descend on the congregation this special Easter Sunday. The Bishop was our esteemed guest. He was about 40. No doubt he received many competing invitations this Easter, but Payne Memorial was the largest and most prosperous church in his district. Accepting this invitation was a no-brainer. He would serve communion.

I had memorized to perfection my Easter verse for the afternoon service. The Bishop was present for the dedication of our new church in the afternoon– right in the middle of the Easter program. *Oh, darn! With this service running long and another later today, Sunday dinner may have to be rushed.* It would be a real shame to hurry such a feast. I prayed for a miracle to forestall the impending tragedy. My godmother had taught me that the Almighty may not come when you want him, but he is always right on time. My prayer, as earnest as any an eight-year-old boy ever mustered, was about to be answered, but not in a manner that I or anyone else could have imagined. Dark storm clouds were gathering and would surely rain on this Easter parade.

As Lizzie took her seat, the Stewardesses rose to dress the altar rail for communion. The music drifted to the foreground as if to shield their work, which paved the way for a second round of prancing and promenading. It was no accident that the offering was positioned to precede the altar call and communion. Had the offering come last, the funds collected would have been greatly diminished.

The altar was dressed. I knew that service would be over once communion was served. Miss Tread would not have to get up and go to the altar rail as communion would be brought to her. Only the Elders, Stewardesses—and Miss Tread—received this honor.

From out of nowhere blustered a sudden storm shattering the apparent solemnness and sanctity of the ritual. In an unfathomable act that was totally out of order, a gussied-up woman whose voice clamored above the congregation like thunder, unleashed an obtuse rant about "…heathens and adulterers in our midst!" We all gasped. The music stopped.

I turned and stretched and with effort could see that it was Ada, Miss Tread's sister-in-law. Ada was a would-be social climber who never got the community stature she desired. I did not like her. She was always trying—and failing—to upstage my mom. I was not sure what all the commotion was about, but I feared it may preempt me from pilfering my last piece of candy, or worse still, lengthen the service.

This was not how service was supposed to go. I knew because there was no entry in the bulletin for tantrums. All crying babies and troublesome youths were sequestered in the basement. There should be no surprises. I looked to the choir loft behind the altar in search of my mother's face. She would know what to do, and she could communicate it with a look. I found her eyes fixed on me, directing me not to move or speak.

Ada's fury continued. The congregation was gripped by a stunned silence, as if in fear of being struck by lightning. Lizzie rose to leave. That is when everyone noticed her among the sea of silk, taffeta, chiffon, linen, perfume, purses, and the sailboat headgear. It was only then that I realized Lizzie must be the object of the darkness gushing from Ada's mouth.

But the storm was about to take an astonishing turn. At that moment, Miss Tread stood up, stepped into the aisle and instructed Lizzie not to move. She then hobbled toward the ranting woman, cane in hand, but menacingly raised in the air like the staff of Moses in *The Ten Commandments*, and said bluntly but loud enough for everyone to hear, "Ada, sit down and shut up!"

Miss Tread whirled around to the Bishop and told him to sit down, too. Some of the ushers started toward her—at least they did until Mr. Tread stirred—all six feet four inches of him—among the trustees seated at the front of the church. I saw my father step into the aisle at the back of the church. As Mr. Tread stood quietly but deliberately, everyone backed away from his wife, and the Bishop stepped away from the altar rail.

Miss Tread spun around and faced the congregants who had not breathed since Ada started her rant. Ada shriveled back into her pew. Time was suspended like a chandelier from the high ceiling and the air crackled with electricity. I had never seen Miss Tread so animated, but in that moment she was Moses descending from Mount Sinai.

Only the handkerchief remained where Miss Tread had been seated seconds before, enjoying the choir and organist as they set a serene air for communion. I reached over and took the last piece of candy, popped it into my mouth and chewed. I chewed for dear life, and then pivoted on the seat to track Miss Tread's steps. The Bishop returned to the lectern, imploring my godmother to sit down and gesturing for the ushers to escort Lizzie from the congregation. Again, Miss Tread whirled around and pointed her cane at the Bishop. "I've got something to say, and I'm going to say it – and I'm going to say it now! I told you to sit down or I'll start with you!...Lizzie, don't you move! Tread (to her husband), I'm OK."

With that she pivoted and continued her trek into the midst of the sanctuary.

"Stand up, Lizzie. Get up. You there, move out of the lady's way...Lizzie, take my seat – go on. That's right, but don't sit down. I want these so-called Christians to take a good look at you."

I struggled with all my might to catch her words as they sliced through the air. Then I caught the scent of Lizzie's expensive perfume. She was standing there, a few feet away from me, just inside my row. I swallowed the last of the candy and listened. It soon became clear to me that Miss Tread was recalling little known and tragic events that had occurred in these people's lives. The Payne Memorial's own anagnorisis was in progress, and that certainly was not in the bulletin.

She moved up and down the aisle, back and forth, her small melodic voice cutting like the sharpest razor. Anyone who dared attempt to sneak out was called to atonement. The newly installed state-of-the-art central air conditioning system had cycled off, so her voice sailed unchallenged through the space.

"Charles, remember when your little girl was in the hospital on the respirator and you couldn't pay for ..."

"Beulah, remember when your Mother's house burned to the ground, and ..."

"James, remember when your hands were crushed at the plant and you had to have emergency surgery? You had no insurance, but your bills were paid?..."

She did not swear. She did not ridicule. But people were sobbing. What mysterious power was she wielding over these pillars of the community? She was more relentless than Jesus challenging the money changers in the temple. As she reeled about pointing that cane at various parishioners, her words were powerful enough to upend tables and overturn chairs.

"Remember those building fund rallies that paid for the air conditioning you ungrateful gluttons are wallowing in today? The intercom and the sound systems? That expensive Conn organ? ..."

A community rally to provide disaster assistance to a flooded neighborhood after a spring thaw (that happened a lot). College or vocational school tuition for someone's son or daughter. Seed money to generate matching funds for an urban renewal project. A community center. Medical equipment. Small business loans that a bank would not touch.

The list went on and on and on. All the pain and heartache of financial uncertainty, illnesses, work-related accidents, fires, and death—even the construction of this huge sanctuary—were presented as if evidence in a public trial. Miss Tread punctuated each show of proof by pointing her cane toward Lizzie – the benefactor – and calling her name, while keeping her eyes fixed on the object of her reproach.

"When you get on your knees to pray tonight before you go to bed, you thank Lizzie for the generosity and compassion that have allowed your sorry asses to be here today!"

This is what those meetings with the tea cakes and the chicory coffee were really all about!

Yes, Miss Tread could raise funds, or lobby the legislature for public policy issues and urban renewal projects. But her most reliable underwriter was the lady who drove that convertible Cadillac. Lizzie was the secret weapon in Miss Tread's arsenal of supporters.

Lizzie was sold to a brothel when she was a toddler in the early 1920's. The Madam who bought her, cared for her and was likely responsible for saving her life. She spent her childhood and adolescence in the care of the Madam, and from that cocoon she emerged as a butterfly—a stunning beauty. She was unable to attend school, because this was a perfect community and Lizzy's circumstances were anything but perfect. Somehow she learned to read and write. She was a whiz at accounting and finance. Lizzie would eventually take over the operation of the brothel, transforming a seedy operation into a multi-million dollar enterprise. Her employees were healthy and had access to the best medical care. They serviced politicians and moguls of industry and commerce throughout the Midwest and the Eastern seaboard. Many were "promoted" to set up "legitimate" businesses and normalized lifestyles. Lizzie even managed to keep organized crime at bay. It would seem that there was an entire underground economy that depended on her intellectual property. Who knew?

And somewhere along that bitter path, Lizzie met my godmother and guardian angel. They struck a secret bargain, and those tea visits were like board meetings where Miss Tread and Lizzie reviewed the needs of the community, discussed the politics of the day, and planned their special interest lobbying strategies for the coming year. With a plan in place, Miss Tread would get busy "laundering" Lizzie's funds into respectable and charitable ventures and services.

"Choir, sing something – something sweet," instructed Miss Tread. "Bishop, you can start the communion."

I hear strains of a familiar hymn sung softly in the background:

> *Come, ye disconsolate, where're ye languish*
> *Come to the mercy seat, fervently kneel*
> *Here bring your wounded hearts*
> *Here tell your anguish*
> *Earth has no sorrow that heaven cannot heal.*

The bishop followed by the pastor left the altar and served the communion elements to the Stewardesses on the front row. But what happened next was yet another singular occurrence that I dare say would not be repeated. Ever.

The Bishop and Pastor moved toward our pew where both knelt and served communion to Miss Tread—*and* to Lizzie.

… May the body and blood of our Lord Jesus Christ keep you unto eternal life…
… May the body and blood of our Lord Jesus Christ keep you unto eternal life…

The honor reserved for the Trustee Board, Stewardesses, and Miss Tread, was extended to Lizzie!

I saw a tear on Lizzy's cheek. Miss Tread gave Lizzie her handkerchief—the magic one that once held my candy treasures. The Bishop and Pastor returned to the altar, to start the communion service for the congregation at large. The ushers started with the last row at the back of the church, and progressed forward row by row, directing people down the center aisle in double lines to the altar rail where they received the sacrament. Congregants returned to their pews by the side aisles. Of course that meant everyone had to pass Lizzie—at least once. This time the air of strutting and preening was replaced by true solemnness and sanctity.

After what seemed like an eternity, everyone was back in their seats and communion was finally served to the trustees. The Bishop lifted his arms, saying, "All rise." The muffled rustle of hundreds of people getting up at once rippled through the sanctuary. But wait.

As the Bishop offered up the benediction, Miss Tread stepped out into the aisle. She stretched out her hand, and Lizzie took it. Miss Tread winked at me to follow. And we three, hand in hand, walked down the center aisle while the parishioners' heads were bowed during the Bishop's prayer.

Despite her unfortunate genesis replete with circumstances over which she had no control, Lizzie forgave her community, her parents, and herself. Her fortuitous partnership with my godmother brought peace and solace to her life. In the process, she transcended her circumstances to offer hope to those ostensibly with better lives than her own. Nowhere have I witnessed anything to rival her extreme virtue and radical generosity.

That day my ideal and predictable life was blown away like so many leaves in the wind. Our perfect community was not so perfect after all. And yet, there were treasures buried there in the rich soil of that American Heartland, and one of those treasures was my godmother.

Gandhi once said, "I like your Christ. I do not like your Christians." I have a feeling Gandhi would have liked my godmother. She was the personification of Christianity. That day she opened my eyes to the concept of paying one's blessings forward. Of course, I did not understand it at the time. From her I learned the importance of understanding why I do what I do. While it is good to do the right thing. It is better to do the right thing for the right reason.

There was an extra plate at Miss Tread's table that Easter Sunday – and dinner was not rushed.

6 Dad

Robert Feldman Harvey, my father, was born November 27, 1915 somewhere in Brazoria County, Texas. His childhood is pretty much a blank slate for me, as he shared almost no information about his childhood. Anything I recall about his origins was told to me by my mother and gleaned from her brief encounter with my father's parents. His mother was a Native American but I do not know the name of her tribe. By the time my parents married, my paternal grandmother had suffered a stroke. She was paralyzed from the waist down and unable to speak. I remember seeing a picture of her in a wheelchair, legs draped in a handwoven blanket. She appeared to be a proud woman whose body had been ravaged by poor health. Her husband stood beside her. I do not know their names. My paternal grandfather was a presiding elder in the African Methodist Episcopal

(A.M.E.) Church, and travelled throughout South Texas overseeing revivals, conducting missionary work, and occasionally providing mentorship to other A.M.E. pastors. Those to whom he provided care and guidance offered primarily chickens, produce, and handmade items as compensation. This infers a rather meager lifestyle for my father and his siblings. At some point the family moved from Brazoria County to Waco, Texas.

My father had four brothers and two sisters, but two of his brothers were deceased before I was born. With the exception of an older brother, my father's siblings remained in Waco until they died. I never understood what kept them anchored in this small remote town distinguished only as home to Baylor University and by its proximity to the ranch owned by President George W. Bush.

Each of Dad's living siblings completed undergraduate college studies by the mid-1930's at Historically Black Colleges and Universities (HBCUs). This would have been considered an outstanding achievement at the time.

My dad and his older brother attended Wiley College in Marshall, Texas. As fate would have it, Granny saw fit to send Mom South for her college education, and enrolled her at Wiley College in the fall of 1936. It was in Marshall that my mother first met my father's older brother. They dated briefly but decided they were better as friends. Due to Granny's legal troubles that year, Mom attended college year-round and in the summer of 1937, she was introduced to my dad by her former beau (my father's older brother). Dad had already graduated from Wiley. He was teaching in the public school system and working on his Master's degree. He and Mom registered for the same debate class. Mom had been a champion debater at Englewood High School in Chicago. She was assigned a seat behind my father in class and could not resist popping his suspenders and goading him into debates in which she delighted in adopting obtuse positions.

"Your friends and neighbors have chosen you…" Thus began the telegrammed draft notice my father received, instructing him to report to military duty in support of World War II. My father mused about the fact that he did not know the "friends and neighbors" who were so prominently called out in the order. Nevertheless, World War II was underway and he was compelled by his fervent patriotism to report for duty in the United States Army. But not before he and my mother were married by the president of Wiley College in June 1942.

At that time, troops were segregated by race. Many black military units were deployed for construction work, building roads and temporary runways, housing, warehousing facilities, and other structures in preparation for the arrival of military personnel. Much of my father's deployment was in the Pacific war zone. He spent many months in the Philippines and New Guinea, leading an operations support unit and attaining the rank of First Lieutenant.

Dad's time in military service was difficult. He once shared that he stopped getting to know people in the service because he would meet someone and the next thing he knew, that person would be dead. He was emotionally scarred by the experience and built walls around his person to protect and shore up himself.

I always suspected the horrors he experienced during the war repressed whatever emotional expression he retained from his inscrutable childhood. Naturally, he did not speak often of his time in the military, and only rarely shared stories about the troops under his command, but his comportment was sufficient to earn an early combat release.

McLennnan Phillip Harvey was my father's younger brother. Uncle Mac was tall, at six feet three inches, and rather stout. He seemed always to be in a good mood, offering positive encouragement to others. He was a jolly prankster of sorts and was extremely generous with his time and acts of goodwill. He was an English professor at Paul Quinn College for two decades, beginning in the 1950's. Uncle

Mac owned the *Waco Messenger*, a black newspaper founded in the 1920's by L. J. Rhone and published by Smith Printing Company. The newspaper and the printing company were housed in the same building on Bridge Street, which was a mecca for African-American business owners in McLennan County. My uncle shepherded the *Waco Messenger* from the 1960's until his death in the 1980's.

Simian James Harvey was my Dad's oldest living brother. Uncle SJ was the only member of the Harvey clan who escaped west and established his home in Los Angeles. He actually attained a Ph.D., and I suspect he found himself professionally "invisible", as were so many college-educated black males in the 30's and 40's. Despite his credentials, he worked for the United States Postal Service until his death in the late 70's. Uncle SJ was also tall, standing six feet four inches, his vocal resonance emulating that of the famous entertainer, Nat King Cole. He was my favorite uncle. I always hoped I would be as tall as he, and develop a deep, resonant voice similar to his. He wore a gentle smile that appeared to be backlit from a movie set as he moved with the grace of Fred Astaire. He and his wife, Gracie, were not blessed with children. I always believed Uncle SJ allowed himself to be trapped by Aunt Gracie, who seemed forever to be competing for a more prominent position within the Harvey clan. For years Aunt Gracie claimed to hold some fabulous senior administrative position with the Los Angeles Independent School District. She bragged to my cousins and me about her important profession. This myth persisted until the afternoon of my Uncle Mac's funeral, wherein my mother summarily defrocked Aunt Gracie, revealing that she was only a cook at an elementary school—and not even the head cook. We never saw Aunt Gracie after that. But the incident sealed my opinion that there was some underlying discontent in Uncle SJ's marriage.

I also knew Dad's older sister, Ella Niece, and his baby sister, Aunt Carrie. Aunt Ella Niece was an extreme introvert, never challenging the authority of her husband, Buford Tatum. She was a schoolteacher in Tatum, Texas for many years, but in the early 1970's, she and her husband built a house in Waco adjacent to Uncle Mac's house. Aunt Carrie, on the other hand, was an extrovert who lived life out loud in the otherwise tranquil community of Waco. She and her husband, Uncle Jack, never had children. I was always uncomfortable around the two of them, feeling there may be something unseemly just below the surface.

Once out of military service, Dad applied to both medical and dental school, knowing that his tuition would be covered by the G.I. Bill. His first choice was medical school, but there was an explosion of veteran applicants during World War II and enrollment was granted on a first-come-first-served basis. The University of Iowa College of Dentistry in Iowa City offered Dad a slot and he took it primarily because it was offered first, but also because it would fund Mom's return to Iowa where Granny was now struggling to care for her terminally ill husband, Grandpa Franklin. Having been rescued and raised by Granny, my mother was anxious to help the only mother she had ever known. (Ironically, Dad was also accepted into medical school two weeks after he committed to dental school.) He remained in dental school an extra year to garner his credentials in oral surgery. Mom's grandfather eventually succumbed to mesothelioma (black lung disease).

Upon graduation in 1953, Dad was recruited aggressively by the town of Waterloo, Iowa due to a shortage of dental services in that community. He used his last dollars to move my mother and their five-year-old daughter to Waterloo. But Dad was not warmly received, as expected, in this northeastern Iowa town. He had been recruited solely on the basis of his academic credentials. Apparently, the city fathers did not know there were African-American graduates from the College of Dentistry at the University of Iowa. In Waterloo there were three major hospitals — Schoitz, Allen, and St. Francis. My father applied for surgical privileges at all three and was promptly denied. Desperately in need of income, Dad established a general dentistry office in Waterloo, where he practiced successfully for 20 years. It was a love-hate relationship, to be sure.

My father was just shy of his 40th birthday when I was born in 1955. Perhaps it was because he was in his mid-50's when I entered high school that there was such a significant generation gap between us. He tried once or twice to play catch with me, but his work schedule was so arduous that he could not be counted on as a reliable playmate. Being a very logical man it seemed odd to me that he became jealous when I found other males to fill that role.

Case in point. Willa Mae was in Mom's Sunday school class. I got the impression that Willa Mae attended Sunday school as a kind of escape from her environment. Mom was Willa Mae's refuge. They became quite close. Willa Mae was 15 years or so older than I, and the only person other than Miss Tread, entrusted with my care. She was very striking in appearance with a strong and rich alto voice and a dry sense of humor. Shortly after enrolling at Iowa State Teachers College, she met and began dating a young man named Charlie. It was important to Willa Mae that Charlie had Dad's approval. Charlie was Dr. Martin Luther King, Jr.'s first cousin. In fact, his resemblance to Dr. King was absolutely remarkable. He also had the aura of actor Billie D. Williams, but most important to me, he was athletic, and Mom and Dad loved him. When Willa Mae babysat, it was okay if Charlie also stopped by. He played ball with me. We wrestled and rolled around on the lawn. I was about five. When Charlie proposed to Willa Mae, I was excited because they wanted me to be the ring bearer. The wedding would be held at The Little Brown Church in the Vale (in Nashua, IA), a popular place for weddings. I rehearsed until had the ring bearer's part down pat. On the day of the wedding, Mom was anxious to leave on time to assure our early arrival. The drive would take about an hour and a half. Curiously, Dad, who was always extremely punctual, dawdled. In fact, because of him, we did not arrive at the church until the wedding was over. Years later, my mother would affirm that my dad was jealous of Charlie's relationship with me. His tardiness that day was no accident. While I am no psychologist, I believe his behavior had a passive-aggressive ring to it.

I never doubted that Dad had a tremendously strong love for his family, but he seemed content to sit across the room reading the newspaper, and only occasionally to dip one corner of the paper to survey the room as if seeking assurance that we were all present and safe.

The house where I lived the first five years of my life was located at the corner of Beech and Sumner in the Rose Hill Addition on the eastside. Dad owned the adjacent lot. This first house was craftsman style and wood framed with dark red brick geometric columns accenting the front porch. On the south, east, and west, the house was cradled by cottonwood trees. A large weeping willow tree formed an oversized umbrella on the eastern property line.

Directly across the street stood Ulysses S. Grant Elementary School, a large turn-of-the-century three-story brick structure surrounded by a public park. I remember the park well, as it served as the safety zone where I daily mounted the back of our large rough collie named Prince. There were pictures of Prince standing on his hind legs and lopping his front paws over Mr. Tread's shoulders. My father rescued Prince from a Special Forces dog pound that trained attack dogs to support the troops during the Korean War. My mother told the story that when she and Dad arrived, they noticed all the dogs were kenneled together, except an oversized rough collie and a Doberman pinscher. These two dogs were isolated to protect the others. Both were trained to never bark, and to attack on cue from simple hand gestures or a single word. Dad was drawn to the isolated pen, which he entered to the shock of the troops guarding the kennel. They were afraid he would be ripped to shreds, but both dogs immediately ran to him and sat at attention in front of him, waiting for his instruction. Dad always had an uncanny way with animals. He romped for a time with both dogs who seemed eager to please him. Finally, he chose the Collie because it appeared less menacing than the Doberman.

Prince allowed me to climb on his back and ride him like a horse. *Lassie* was a popular TV show at the time, starring a highly intelligent rough collie who often came to the aid of the costar, a little boy named Timmy. I often imagined myself as Timmy when riding Prince around the park. He would walk the perimeter of the park one time, return me to my front yard and sit. At that point it would be impossible to move him. He never barked or knocked me down, but he let me know when playtime was over.

We kept Prince until we moved into town. Dad gave him to a farmer in Black Hawk County because he could not stand the idea of Prince chained up in a small backyard. A collie needed room to roam freely. I was devastated and cried for days over the loss of my protector and friend.

The dining room in the craftsman home was separated from the living room by two geometric wooden columns, mimicking the brick columns on the front porch, but framed two bookcases. Just inside the dining room in the corner stood a large wooden pedestal supporting a huge unabridged *Oxford Dictionary of the English Language*. My father built a wooden stepstool so I could safely climb up and turn the pages. This dictionary was too large for one person to hold and manipulate the pages at the same time. So it rested nobly on its pedestal, ever ready to explain the pronunciation, connotation, etymology, and context of every word in the English language. We had two full sets of encyclopedias on the shelves of those built-in bookcases, but I knew, even as a 4-year-old, that the Oxford dictionary reigned supreme.

One Saturday my father instructed me to go to the dictionary and find the largest word. I climbed the stepstool and dutifully surveyed the printed landscape before me. With both hands I carefully turned the pages in search of the largest word. I eventually gave up and looked around with bewilderment to summon my father's assistance. He walked up beside me and turned to the word *no*. Having learned to read at Miss Tread's dining room table when I was three years old, I read well enough to know that the word *no* was not the largest word in the dictionary, and I told him so. He smiled and put his finger over the definition of the word and said, "The day you learn to use this word to frame the beginning, middle and end of a conversation, without the need to explain or debate its usage, will be the day you become a man."

Another 20 years would come and go before I understood what he meant. I remember being given a command by one of my co-workers, to which I simply responded, "No." I spoke the word without inflection or sarcasm. But I remember the facial expression of the person who barked the order, and it was immediately clear that the conversation had been closed by my simple statement. In that moment I understood my father's prediction, and I smiled, realizing I had claimed my manhood.

It is a not-so-subtle irony, that the word *no* loomed large in Dad's own life. He heard it three times after applying for surgery privileges at three hospitals in Waterloo. He heard it too many times to count when he embarked upon a relatively simple plan to construct a suitable home for his family. And fortunately for all concerned, Dad heard and *felt* Mr. Tread's resounding *No!* when my sister was sexually assaulted.

On the eve of my first day of kindergarten I remember my father lifting me and standing me on a stool so I could pick the pencil I would take to class the next day. Looking me directly in my eyes he explained that I was a member of the Harvey family, and that every member of the family had a job. His job and that of my mother was to provide a shelter and food—and heat in the winter time. My job as a member of the family would begin the next day, my first day of school. He told me that my job was to go to school…

> "… And to learn something while there. If there's something you don't understand, politely raise your hand and get the attention of your teacher.

State your question and listen to the answer. If you are unsatisfied with the answer or it fails to fully address your question, come home and ask your mother or me. We will try to offer a satisfactory answer. If you are still confused, we will accompany you to meet with your teacher and work with him or her to find an answer that fully addresses your interests. It is perfectly okay to ask questions. After all, your job is to learn as much as possible."

Naturally, I thought my classmates received similar instructions from their parents, but I was very wrong. Most of my peers knew they had to attend school, but they did not seem to know why they were there. School for them was a structured extension of playtime. But I was on a quest for knowledge as I believed this was my job as a member of the Harvey family. I suffered astigmatism in both axes in both eyes, and was extremely nearsighted. This problem with my vision was caught early and I was fitted with black, horn-rimmed glasses. This mask earned me the nickname of "Professor", a label I would bear through high school, not as a pejorative, but as an accurate characterization of the seriousness I attached to learning. It became more of a thumbs-up acknowledgment from my peers of my intellect and sense of social justice.

During the summer of 1960, my family moved from the idyllic Rose Hill community to a house on Lane Street in a neighborhood close to downtown Waterloo but still on the eastside. When we moved, my only concern was losing Prince.

***

The sayings my dad repeated over and over, day in and day out, as if barking military orders, drove me nuts. One of his favorites was, "Pay attention to your environment!" These words seemed to echo around the room, in the car, in the grocery store or wherever we happened to be. I cringed each time he lobbed this curious directive in the air and it landed at my feet like a live grenade that failed to explode. He rarely sat down to discuss the concepts behind his counsel, preferring instead that my understanding come through my own personal experience.

If anyone mentioned a preference for a particular fruit, my father would show up with a bushel of that fruit—more than *anyone* could possibly eat. I was extremely fond of Nabisco Fig Newton cookies. About twice a year I would have a craving for them, and Dad would go out and buy the largest bag he could find. No surprise—that was his way. Unfortunately, he was insensitive to the uniqueness I attached to the Nabisco brand and would show up with some generic, off-brand product. I could tell by the quantity that he was attempting to demonstrate his care and concern, but eating those off-brand "Fig Newton" cookies was like chewing wet cardboard. I did not have the heart to throw them out or ask him for the real deal. For years I suffered, chewing and swallowing those tasteless cookies because I knew they were offered with love. During my middle school years I became adept at not eating but disposing of the tasteless treats all the same, while reassuring Dad that I had consumed them with joy.

The summer following sixth grade and preceding my entrance into middle school was free of obligations and projects. I planned to fill my days building roads and bridges in the dirt with my brand-new set of Tonka trucks, looking forward to my adventures. However, on the first Monday of summer vacation my father entered my bedroom at 6 a.m. and instructed me in that certain tone of his to get dressed and meet him at the car in the next 15 minutes. Without protest I put on the seersucker shorts and matching shirt laid out for me the night before. I tied up my tennis shoes and ran to the car where my father was waiting. We drove in silence to his downtown office, which was located on the top floor of Black's Department Store, Waterloo's version of Macy's. Directly across the street was the Sear's Business School. Dad parked the car and escorted me across the street into the business school, where he registered me for typing classes. This was certainly not an activity that supported playing in the mud with my Tonka trucks. But I did not protest, primarily out of self-preservation.

Classes were scheduled Monday through Friday from 7 until 11 a.m. For the next eight weeks my routine would be to meet Dad at the car promptly at 6:15 a.m., dressed and ready for a day of instruction. It would take all the courage I could muster as a 12-year-old to enter that classroom. It was packed with 17-year-old girls forced to take this class and get a passing grade to make up for the incompletes they received the previous school year. These girls were pissed! It was a hostile environment. But I liked school.

Despite feeling intimidated, I picked a seat in the center of first row in the classroom, and ignored the sneers and baffled looks from the angry girls. Promptly at 7 a.m. a scary figure, dressed in black entered the classroom. Like my Great Aunt Jesse, this woman also resembled The Wicked Witch of the West in *The Wizard of Oz*. She was a no nonsense stickler for perfection. I quickly endeared myself to her, becoming one her favorites, as I found touch typing to be fun. Perhaps I excelled at typing because I developed strength in my fingers from hours of piano practice. To the chagrin of the girls, I attained the highest speed and accuracy in the class, easily typing at least 80 words per minute with no errors. I looked forward to those 7 to 11 a.m. sessions, challenging myself each day to increase my speed.

My enrollment at the Sear's Business School proved invaluable during my college studies. I could not write fast enough to keep up with my brain, but I could type like a madman. Besides my handwriting was atrocious, illegible at times, even to me. So I got in the habit of typing up my notes, and embellishing them from my memory of the lectures and from my textbook readings. This is where touch typing (not needing to look at one's fingers while typing) became my weapon of choice. In the 1980's when word processors and personal computers emerged, my typing skills again placed me ahead of the curve.

Once again I discovered a method to Dad's madness. I forgave him eventually for interfering with my summer Tonka-truck adventures. Although I slowly learned to trust his wisdom and believed I would eventually understand his lessons, his methods were difficult to endure.

A recurring lesson came with his insistence that I accompany him on various shopping trips. I had to dress up, like him. The rules were simple. Be seen, but not heard. Pay attention, but do not speak or ask questions.

I knew the script by heart, as well as the action notes that accompanied the words. My father would enter a store with steadfast intention. He knew what he wanted to buy and he knew how much he was willing to pay. As if on cue, a store attendant would approach and speak the lines, "Good morning, sir. May I help you?" My father would reply, "That remains to be seen."

Without fail, the sales attendant would flash a bewildered look, and I would frantically search for the proverbial hole in the floor. But obedient to my instructions I did not move, look up at my father or ask questions. I found a spot on the floor and fixed my stare there as my imaginary anchor. This was permitted. The sales attendant would invariably take the bait and continue the pointless conversation, "Well, sir, it's my job to be of assistance." Dad would snap back, "It has yet to be determined whether you are qualified to perform that service." By then I would be excavating desperately that hole into which I wanted to jump and bury myself, but I dared not reveal my fight or flight impulse. "I would prefer to speak with someone of authority within this establishment. Someone who need not ask anyone's permission." The sales attendant's eyes would move up and to the right as if in deep contemplation. My father would seize the opportunity and say, "I wish to speak to the person you are thinking about right now." At this point a manager would be summoned and my father would state in a declarative manner what he wanted, and would inquire about the price. If the price point was not within the parameters he established for himself, he would simply say, "Thank you, but I'm no longer interested." Should the manager attempt to negotiate or convince my father to buy with the usual spiel, my father would look that manager dead his eyes and say, "It's my money and I don't have to spend it here!" With that he would pivot 180 degrees and head for the nearest exit. That would be my cue to follow.

I dreaded these command excursions. He never explained his behavior and never apologized for it. I knew him to be a stickler for protocol and decorum. So I did not understand his terse treatment of salespeople, but I dared not interrogate his intentions. I remained in a quandary over these sessions until I found myself 40 years later attempting to buy a dishwasher at a Home Depot Expo Design Center. After asking several questions about functional design and quality of competing high-end brands and being repeatedly told by the salesperson, "I don't know," I wheeled around and said, "Then why are you wasting my time?" The sales attendant backed up a few feet and started to nervously explain that this was not his department and that he was substituting for the regular specialist. I began to smirk, struggling to hold back gut-busting laughter, which only further intimidated the salesperson. I put up my hands and waved them around trying to calm the terrified attendant. I realized in that moment that I was channeling my father. *OMG! I have become him*, I thought to myself, smiling inside.

***

Dad was a man with a plan. He invested in several undeveloped lots in east Waterloo. He moved our craftsman house from 904 Beech at Sumner Streets to one of his vacant lots, renovated the house and leased it. Next he planned to build a house on the Beech Street lot, but the new structure would make full use of the adjacent lot, which Dad also owned. He estimated that we would live on Lane Street no more than a year—two at the outside. But a never-ending stream of No's would confine us to Lane Street for the next decade.

Grave obstacles presented themselves right from the start. The Waterloo city planning commission would not approve Dad's building plans. The city's position was that "this is too nice a house to build on the eastside." But it was Dad's land and money, and Dad's right to use both in any legal manner of his choosing. After months of obstruction and bureaucratic red tape, my father obtained the permits necessary to move forward with his project, entering into a heroic struggle to build the house of his choice on the site of his choice. Dad would hire no fewer than three general contractors, white and black. As if the fight with the city were not stressful enough, his contractors challenged him on the orientation of the structure, the foundation elevation, building materials, electrical wiring and various construction standards.

The plans for the split-level house called for 1,582 square feet of living space with three bedrooms and two baths. The brick and wood structure would be positioned at a 45 degree angle straddling the two lots. Preparation of the construction site began finally in 1961.

As the lots were located at the bottom of two hills, winter thaws and spring rains caused regular floodwaters to settle there. Dad insisted that the ground be built up by some 8 to 10 feet to counteract the flow of water and support the split-level design. City's objection: This was an excessive and unnecessary measure.

Dad insisted on a poured concrete basement, complete with 9-inch French drains to mitigate basement flooding. City's objection: Cinderblock basement walls were the current construction standard.

Dad demanded higher than standard insulation for the exterior walls and the attic to protect against the harsh winters and insulate the dwelling from the extremes of cold and hot weather. City's objection: No need for higher than standard insulation.

Dad insisted on a certain number of 220 electrical circuits to support the heating and cooling systems, and appliances, and a certain number of 110 electrical outlets on every exterior wall. City's objection: Too many 220 circuits and too many electrical outlets.

The general contractors also objected to: Double-paned, thermal glass windows throughout the structure; the quality of solid wood and thermally insulated exterior doors; and the installation of white oak floors, cabinetry, and wood trim throughout the structure.

In the summer of 1968, seven years after the construction project was launched, Dad asked me to visit the construction site daily and report on the progress. I should pay close attention to the standards as defined in the building plans. I was excited to be included in the project, but I had no idea this project had been underway for six years. I thought it was just beginning. To my great advantage, a 13-year-old boy could not be perceived by contractors as a threat. I was able to observe the construction closely without arousing suspicion. Miss Tread, still lived at the other end of the block from the site, which made her home a kind of convenient staging area/construction office/diner.

Dad and I visited the construction site one evening, after hours. The workers had left for the day. Dad was dressed in a business suit and a trench coat. We discovered that hollow core double front doors had been installed instead of the solid wood doors specified in the plans. Dad returned to his car to get a screwdriver, which he used together with his bare hands to rip the doors from their hinges and throw them into the front yard.

Although the third contractor managed to finish the project, it was during his tenure that all the copper piping was stolen because he failed to secure the property. We strongly suspected that this guy was in cahoots with the copper thieves.

When we finally moved into the new house in the summer of 1970, all who visited from near and far deemed it a premier property. Although I was still unaware of the significance of our new home to my parents and the community, I was delighted to wake up each morning inside an issue of *Architectural Digest*.

***

As I look back on my relationship with my father, I can recall three critical junctures when his understanding, advice, or elucidation could have made all the difference in my life. These were times when I wanted and needed to hear my father's perspective, but he was unwilling or unable to *talk it out*. Perhaps this was emblematic of the generational differences between us. Perhaps it was due to the horrors he witnessed during his military service. Or perhaps it was simply his way. Whatever the reason, it seemed to me that the more challenging and difficult the situation, the more deafening was his silence.

The first instance came on the heels of my experience as a delegate to the Iowa American Legion Hawkeye Boys State Camp. This was an outstanding honor. The Boys State objective was to instruct young men about city, county, and state government during a weeklong conference devoted to "learning by doing." Over 500 delegates represented Iowa's *diversity* of heritage and culture. The organization prided itself on affording young men friendships with other Boy's State "citizens", many of whom would become lifelong friends. My mother urged me to run for elected office. My heart wasn't in it, but I became a candidate to please her. I had to rally a mock campaign office, surrogates, and platform from among the assemblage of some 30 or so peers in my assigned camping region. I lost the election, but I did make several new acquaintances. I also entered the talent competition, which I won by a landslide with my performance of a Burt Bacharach classic, "A House is Not a Home." I didn't really understand the lyrics, but I loved the haunting melody and construction of the musical composition.

Thinking back on that performance it seems really out of place for me to have been singing this song of longing and romance to a large audience of teenage boys. But I didn't worry about that – it was incumbent upon me to win something, and this was a victory I was confident I could snag. When I finished I was met with a deafening silence for about five seconds. Then suddenly the space exploded with the wild applause of 500 male teenagers and about 50 adult staffers. No doubt about it – I had an amazing voice, I knew how to use it, and I sold the hell out of that song.

My campaign organization celebrated exuberantly. Their candidate had publicly crushed the opposition (regardless of not having won an elected office); everyone else knew who their candidate was; and I was a star for the rest of the conference. (I was one of only a handful of black persons present. Remember this was 1970). As a result of my celebrity, I became friends that week with one young man in particular. He was the son of a powerful state senator from Sioux City, over 200 miles from Waterloo. At the time there was no Internet, of course, and no affordable long-distance calling plans. So we agreed to become pen pals, exchanging written correspondence on a weekly basis. Upon returning home, I began to uphold my end of this bargain, and each week for the next six months he and I exchanged letters. During the first month of correspondence we discovered we shared the same feelings of isolation. Both our fathers were prominent and influential men, and afforded identities and lifestyles imagined by a public that did not know them personally. Those assumed identities were forced upon each of us – their sons. The public thought they knew us too, but we were only isolated figures, living in our fathers' shadows. This shared pain strengthened the psychological and emotional bonds between us. Being teenagers, our vocabularies were too immature and clumsy to artfully articulate our shared angst. Nevertheless, our crude correspondence proceeded to examine our experiences and innermost personal feelings with the hope that we could find comfort in one another's unfiltered expressions. Neither of us had ever contemplated a romantic connection – straight or gay.

Unfortunately my pen pal's father intercepted one of our letters. The senator apparently misinterpreted the expressed thoughts as the early formation of some sort of deviant behavior. He was furious. Tracing down my address, he threw his son in the car one Saturday and drove to Waterloo, arriving early Saturday afternoon just as my father returned home from his customary half-day at the office. The doorbell rang. My father answered the door. My pen pal's father was visibly shocked to see a black family living in a stunning residence, but he had little time working through his cognitive dissonance, as his conversation with my father was brief. He was on a mission to rescue his son's moral character. I don't remember his exact words, but I recall the senator shaking what appeared to be a handwritten letter at my father who took it, read it, and continued their verbal exchange for a few moments more. The whole episode lasted less than ten minutes. My father shut the door and came to find me. He did not yell, but he had "that look" on his face, signaling he was dead serious. My father asked me if I knew the Sioux City boy, and where we had met. I promptly told him he had been part of my campaign organization at Boys State the previous summer.

I did not think there was anything nefarious in the correspondence. Our only intention was to share our mutual angst. And I did not know why I was forbidden to ever contact the young man again. All I knew was that my father stood before me, shaking one of the letters at me (I did not know whether it was my friend's or mine), ordering me to cease and desist. It was a decree. It was not up for discussion. In fact, it was never mentioned again.

Unable to ask questions or discuss the matter, I was forced to try to make sense of this situation on my own. I deduced from my father's tone and pained expression that there was something horribly taboo – evil even – about exploring private sentiments with another person. Of course, this was an erroneous and unhelpful deduction, but it was the one I made. Sadly, I feel certain that my father also went away with an erroneous interpretation of the incident.

As I approached draft age, the conundrum of patriotism vis-à-vis my fear and disdain for the atrocities of war would again strain my relationship with my father. It was during the Vietnam War. The evening news on all three networks (NBC, ABC, and CBS) broadcast horrific images of despondent Indochinese (Vietnam, Laos, Cambodia) civilians either setting themselves on fire, or being executed summarily. These nightly horrors were framed by commercials for Shake & Bake, AJAX kitchen cleaner, and Billy Graham telethon trailers. Eventually, college campus protests swelled across the nation as public support for the war began to sour, and suspicions fermented regarding the true motives for sacrificing our young men in a land few had ever heard of. Tough questions raised before Congress, and posed to the new president, Richard Milhouse Nixon, went unanswered. Civilian and military death tolls became as familiar as sports league statistics. Even in the farming and manufacturing community of Waterloo, a steady trickle of death notices seeped through our neighborhood like the flu. I observed once-vibrant young men – the same age as my sister – who returned from that war a mere shadow of their former selves. The sad and haunting dullness in their eyes was a worrisome thing, whether or not they were physically wounded.

Although I had no deep understanding of the protests or the riots, I was terrified about the prospect of being drafted. With each passing month, I struggled to imagine whether or not I would become another casualty of this incomprehensible war, as many young men fled to Canada to avoid conscription. If I should decide to follow them when my time came, exactly how would I go about it? What were the legal implications? Since there was so much at stake, almost no information sources, and so much I didn't know, I counted on my father to help me find information and evaluate my options. He was still my tried and true sage. Dad refused to have this conversation with me. To his way of thinking, I must serve, if drafted, because service was noble. Otherwise, I would be shirking the responsibilities of American citizenship. End of story. There was no discussion. As he shut down, the vacuous silence between us was filled by a haunting ballad recorded by Roberta Flack, expressing the nightmare that played as a loop in my head. The song was entitled, *The Ballad of Sad Young Men*.

> *Sing a song of sad young men, glasses full of rye*
> *All the news is bad again, kiss your dreams goodbye...*
>
> *All the sad young men, drifting through the town*
> *Drinking up the night, trying not to drown...*
>
> *All the sad young men, choking on their youth*
> *Trying to be brave, running from the truth...*
>
> *Misbegotten moon shine for sad young men*
> *Let your gentle light guide them home again*
> *All the sad, sad, sad, young men*

Of course, I cannot be absolutely sure how my father would have reacted had I escaped to Canada, but it would probably have been the end of our relationship. As it happened, in 1969 the Selective Service System began conducting lotteries, using birthdates to determine the order of call to military service. When I reached draft age, my birthdate fell low enough on the list to virtually assure that I would not be called. And so, the question of military service became a moot one, saving for the time being, at least, my relationship with my father.

Nonetheless, I was not entirely unscathed by the war. On May 4th the following year, on the campus of Kent State University, the nation's angst would reach a crescendo as the National Guard killed four students and wounded nine, protesting Nixon's bombing of Cambodia. Inexplicably, the war seemed to be turned inside out as our military appeared to slaughter our own on American soil. Sentiments soured against the troops fighting in Indochina as some four million students – an unimaginable number, at the time – staged walkouts across the nation's college and university campuses. Blind hatred seared all the "sad young men" who had been snatched from their families by a mandatory draft and manipulated like marionettes.

The last draft call was on December 7, 1972, and the authority to induct expired in 1973. Registration with the Selective Service System was suspended in 1975. Conservative estimates place the number of war-related deaths in Vietnam at nearly a million, including 84,000 children, 655,000 adult males, 143,000 adult females, and more than 65,000 allied troops. Over 58,000 American soldiers died in combat. These figures do not include those physically wounded or psychologically traumatized.

Years later, I would encounter two Veterans of this enigmatic conflict: Tony, an affable, professional baseball umpire whose family and childhood friends had suffered during his deployment in the jungles of Indochina; and Will, a manic Marine Corp test pilot, who self-medicated his post-traumatic stress disorder (PTSD) and "escaped" his living nightmare, hosting lascivious parties. As I detail in chapter eleven, my interaction with both men would leave indelible marks on me, and (especially in the case of the test pilot) would darken the journey toward my medical crisis.

The final strain in my relationship with my father came in my mid-30's after I contracted a serious case of food poisoning and was hospitalized for eight days. Lying there without much to do, I began to reflect on the mystery of Dad's family.

As a child my father took the family on three and four-week cross-country trips every summer. I heard "See the USA in your Chevrolet" on TV and believed everyone had the freedom and resources to take such excursions. During these trips, my father's alter ego emerged. He became the jolly traveler, ready for adventure. We travelled throughout the southwest and western United States. Wherever we went, we managed somehow to make stops in Los Angeles and Waco. This is how I came to know my paternal uncles and aunts.

Curiously, when the Harvey siblings got together, there would come a time, usually before dinner, when they would leave their spouses and children for several hours. They would then reappear and rejoin us as if believing their absence had gone unnoticed. As I entered my young adult years I often reflected on how strange it was that there was never a discussion about these mysterious sibling conferences. It was as though they were members of a secret kids' club.

Although my father visited his siblings and kept in close touch with them, I thought it also strange that we never discussed or attended family reunions. When there is a vacuum of information, it is not uncommon to fill the void with negative assumptions and imaginings that may have little to do with reality. But I reasoned, if he were proud of his parentage and his childhood, why would he conceal this information?

Such were my musings as my parents walked into my hospital room. Now was as good a time as any to challenge Dad about his background. I could always ask Mom anything. She might take a moment to reflect on my question, but never failed to answer to the best of her ability. I asked Dad if he had been physically or mentally abused as a child. He seemed shocked by my query, but did his best to maintain a stoic facade. My mom looked at him as if wondering how he would respond, but she did not say a word. I pressed him on the issue, pointing out that I had no reference for his branch of the family tree. I did not know the extent to which that history may impact me. If I did not know anything about his parentage or childhood, then I could not know myself. My father listened patiently as I made my case, but simply responded, "There is no reason to discuss our family experience because we (his brothers and sisters) were all present." What a bizarre response. That was it. I had reached my breaking point. Maybe they were all hatched just before they entered college. Seeing that he appeared to be mildly traumatized by my interest, I assured him that he had no worries, because I would *never* seek to understand him or that part of the family ever again! By now all of his siblings were deceased, so there was no one else to entertain my questions. I often hoped that a time would come when we could revisit this conversation, but it was not to be. He was as suborn as I was. Although we continued to greet each other with pleasantries, this exchange ended any meaningful communication between us.

During one of the first weekends of my fall semester at the University of Iowa, a banquet was organized in Waterloo in honor of Dad. This was not surprising since Dad had been quite active in the community after establishing his dental practice. Most notably he served two terms as a member of the Board of Directors of the Independent School District of Waterloo from 1967 until 1973. During this period, the general social unrest sweeping the nation made its way to Waterloo. High school students began to protest social, political, and educational marginalization. Like their counterparts around the country, the students clashed with the agents of the status quo, aiming to claim the full benefits of United States citizenship. I now believe Dad's motivation for seeking elected office was to impart the wisdom he acquired through his personal battles against racial discrimination. He rejected the notion that people should see themselves as victims. He believed positive change could be inspired and achieved by standing firm in one's accomplishments, and demanding respect in the face of obstruction and discrimination. My father's personal and professional persistence garnered him a position of leadership within the black and white communities. As a model of perseverance, he garnered the respect, if not the admiration, of his contemporaries.

I asked if I should come home to attend, but I was told to stay at school. When I called home a day after the event to inquire about how things went, Mom said the banquet was hosted by the chiefs of staff at those same hospitals that had refused to grant Dad surgical privileges 20 years earlier. She told me Dad was in Los Angeles. This came as a shock. I asked if Uncle SJ was okay, assuming only a medical emergency could account for a sudden trip to southern California. My mother assured me Uncle SJ was in good health. She explained further that Dad was in California to take the state dental board exam. He would be flying to Houston the next week to take the same exam for the state of Texas. I was bewildered by this rash of activity until Mom explained what happened the previous evening. The banquet was the brainchild of the chiefs of staff at Schoitz, Allen, and St. Francis hospitals, each of whom had been residents when Dad applied for surgical privileges. Apparently those three doctors had wrestled for two decades with this overt act of racial discrimination. They sought to right this wrong by presenting Dad with framed documents, affirming his surgical privileges at each of the three hospitals. Mom said Dad accepted the awards, came home, and threw them on the dining room table, announcing he was "getting the hell out of this Godforsaken state." Dad passed both state board exams, and within the year my family left Iowa, ending his "medical experiment" north of the Mason Dixon line. Promising he would "never to be buried in the state of Iowa", my father returned to his native Texas to be close to his surviving siblings. In Dallas, Dad opened a dental practice, which he operated successfully until his retirement in 1993.

As far as the community could determine, we left Waterloo suddenly, and only three years after moving to the house on Beech Street. Rumors began to circulate among my family's detractors that Dad had suffered financial ruin. What else could explain why he would desert such a fine home? After all, this was the same home he had waged a marathon battle to build. In the small minds of these people, financial ruin was the only plausible explanation.

The resistance Dad endured to build the Beech Street house seemed even more ridiculous when I saw our Dallas home, which was situated on a half-acre bordered by a wooded creek. The 4,000 square-foot house was about 60 percent larger than our former residence, and infinitely more elegant, featuring: an all-brick exterior; six-foot French windows on all sides; and a terraced backyard, boasting 600 pink, white, and red azaleas, complete with lighting perfect for evening entertaining. The home was stately and elegant throughout. If my parents had attempted to build our Dallas home in east Waterloo, they might have been exiled.

As she was privy to the false reports of Dad's financial ruin, Miss Tread devised a clever plan to quell the rumors. She handpicked a couple from Payne Memorial A.M.E. Church and encouraged them to pay us a visit in Dallas. Although my parents knew this couple for some 20 years, they were not close friends. The wife was the lead soprano in the choir—and the church gossip. I was summoned home for the weekend from the University of Texas to assist in hosting them. They were giddy and gushing in my parents' company. The husband kept his camera on a tether around his neck, and spent his time taking pictures of his wife, posing inside our home and outside among the azaleas. My parents took them to several elegant restaurants where they dined on scrumptious steak and delectable seafood entrées—and took pictures. I observed all this and for the life of me, could not figure out why these people were visiting us. After a long weekend, the couple returned to Waterloo to report on their fabulous visit with the Harvey's. Their pictures and hyperbolic accounts of our home and Dad's suite of offices finally put to rest the rumors of Dad's financial demise. Miss Tread strikes again.

A few years later, Miss Tread passed away quietly. My parents and I flew to Waterloo to attend her funeral. We intentionally limited our interaction with the locals, preferring to remain quietly in our hotel. With my godmother's passing there was no reason to return to Waterloo ever again.

Despite the differences and the distance between us, I learned so much from my dad. I have to admit that although his technique was arcane and completely unwelcome in my youth, I came to appreciate his efforts to impart his wisdom to me. I learned to connect cause and effect—the consequences of one's actions or failure to act. His lessons and edicts imprinted on my brain became my shield against arrows discharged by hidden agendas, jealousy, and mischief-making. As I witnessed how he negotiated the vicissitudes of his life with dignity and determination, I gained tremendous wisdom and a sense of curiosity about life. We certainly had our differences, but whether he was the man across the room, the jolly traveler with an inscrutable past, or the patriotic military man barking orders to a reluctant son, there can be no doubt he was unequivocal in his love and devotion to his family.

7 SANDRA

Surprise. Shock. Bewilderment. I felt all this and more. It was the first week of November 2009, and this was the last place I expected to be on this day and at this time in my life. The assembled mourners were surprised I was introduced as the brother of the deceased, Sandra Louise Harvey. As I rose to address the congregation of St. Paul's Episcopal Church in Dallas and the assembled friends and acquaintances, I felt lightheaded – as if I was floating – like the feeling I got sometimes after roller skating. I forced myself to shake off that uneasy tension so that I could give a eulogy for my only sibling. Taking my position at the lectern, I surveyed the crowd once more. Only a few faces were familiar to me. There was my cousin Bettye Harvey Smith and her husband, Walter. Sitting next to them was my Uncle Jack, the widower of my late Aunt Carrie. Further back in the crowd were three friends and members of my parents' church, St. Paul A. M. E. Also present was the president of the Southeast Dallas Business and Professional Women's Club.

I was acutely aware that this congregation believed themselves to be intimately familiar with my sister. They knew the care with which she served the children's ministry. They knew she was a capable musician. For her services she was extremely admired and loved by this community. But they could not know how Sandra came to be such a brilliant talent at the keyboard or the extent to which her brilliance had been a source of anguish, frustration, and, yes, disappointment to those who knew her best – her family.

> "Good morning, my name is Reginald Harvey. I am the younger brother of Sandra Harvey, the person whose life we have assembled to memorialize. First, I would like to thank the members of St. Paul's Episcopal Church for providing a safe haven for my sister over the past decade. I am glad to learn that in the last years of her life she found a home for her interests in children's outreach and for her musical talent. I'm certain many of you were astonished by her mastery of organ pedagogy. Finding her way to this congregation, I have no doubt that she bashfully volunteered to assist or substitute in the role of organist, and proceeded to astound those present with her amazing talent. There is a simple explanation for this.
>
> "Sandra not only attended the University of Minnesota School of Music, but also she was the student of Heinrich Fleischer, head of the Organ Department at the University and master instructor at Juilliard. In earlier years she won several regional and national piano competitions whose renown rivaled the internationally famous Van Cliburn Competition held in Fort Worth, Texas. She performed with the Minnesota Symphony among other regional orchestras and ensembles. Despite her savant-like musical prowess, she never leveraged her extraordinary talent into a career,

preferring to quietly blend into the white noise of the world around her.

"For years at a time, she would not touch a piano or organ. We, her family, never knew what initiated these periods or what brought them to a precipitous end. Nevertheless, one fine day, without warning, Sandra would casually sit down at a keyboard, and flawlessly toss off a sonata or concerto as easily as she might toss a salad. Satisfied, she would hop up from the bench with a childish smile, oblivious to the shock and awe of those who witnessed her display."

I could tell by the looks on people's faces that they were perplexed by my words. They were not privy to the conduct Sandra's family ascribed uniquely to her. My remarks were not lengthy, but I was careful to express my gratitude for the kindnesses they had shown my sister during her years among them.

As I returned to my seat, I began a mental perusal of Sandra's difficult life, details that could not be shared in remarks presented at a memorial service. My thoughts took me immediately to 1962. I was only seven years old then, but I recalled a certain event as clearly as if I were watching a movie. The screening was a jumble of flashbacks, revelations, and social contradictions – all rolling simultaneously in both slow-motion and fast-forward. The behavior of the protagonist (my father) contradicted his image as the quiet man behind his newspaper seated across the room.

I saw my godfather, Mr. Tread, restraining Dad in a bear hug, wrestling him to the floor in the entryway of our home. I could smell the leather case holding Dad's World War II Army revolver, and hear that hardened leather case hitting the tile floor. Mr. Treadwell and my father, my mother, and my sister, appeared in three discrete frames as I watched, standing on the edge of the living room carpet, somehow separated from the scene by an invisible wall.

My sister stood alone, sobbing uncontrollably; my mother stood off to the side, frozen in place, neither speaking nor offering comfort to Sandra; and my godfather and my father were writhing on the floor in a desperate struggle as my father grappled for the revolver case while trying to get back on his feet and leave the house.

I now know this traumatic scene ensued as moments earlier, my 15-year-old sister revealed she and her "boyfriend" were expecting a child. Of course, I was oblivious to the context of the unfolding drama, but the 11th commandment in the Harvey household was: no dating until the age of 16. Sandra had broken this sacred decree. Evidently pressured by our father, Sandra disclosed the name of the "boyfriend." My parents knew the unsanctioned, would-be "son-in-law" to be a miscreant and parolee infamous for having fathered a number of children in the community. It would be another decade or so before I learned of the sinister plot to ensnare my sister, and induce this crisis for our family.

At the time I found my mother's behavior odd, as she offered comfort neither to my sister nor my father, preferring instead to stand catatonic, apart from the rest, staring blankly.

Sometime during this same year—before or after the drama erupted, I do not remember which—Dad came to my school, removed me from class and took me to the hospital. It was an adventure to spend time in the waiting room of a hospital. In those days children rarely were allowed into a patient's room, but ice cream and candy suckers were my reward for patiently waiting. What I did not know at the time was that my mother had been admitted for an emergency abortion and complete hysterectomy, made necessary due to an ectopic pregnancy (the fetus was developing in one of her fallopian tubes). Either surgery or the continued pregnancy would have been considered life-threatening in 1962.

Decades later it clicked that my mother's health crisis occurred around the time my parents learned of my sister's pregnancy. I suspect my mother's deafening silence was due either to the trauma that she had just learned of her own pregnancy, or that she had recently endured the emergency abortion and hysterectomy, and was coming to terms with it all. Either way, juxtaposing her daughter's pregnancy with her own situation, *and* witnessing her husband on the floor scuffling with my godfather, could have been sufficient to induce in her a state of shock.

In those days a pregnant teen could be banned from attending school, as a means of protecting the other students from an improper influence. In Waterloo, a girl could not return to school after giving birth, presumably for the same reason. In fact, there was an entire industry involved with "helping" families of pregnant teenage girls. In the decades between World War II and Roe v. Wade, 1.5 million faceless young women were secretly sent to homes for unwed mothers and coerced into giving up their babies for adoption. The social norm of that period held a pregnant teen to be a reflection of failed parenting skills, low morals, and low class. Things like that simply did not happen in "good" families. Surrendering to social norms and the attending guilt and shame, my parents sent Sandra to a "maternity home" – a boarding school for unwed mothers in Des Moines, 110 miles away. Thus my sister joined the ranks of the 1.5 million casualties of the social norm.

As a teenager, I managed to uncover bits and pieces of this story (families did not discuss such things openly in those days). The offender was reportedly very handsome and engaging, traits he used to his advantage in various capers and cons. Sandra knew only that he paid attention to her, and she was convinced he loved and was devoted only to her. Unfortunately, the young man was paid to woo my sister as part of a scheme to embarrass my father. The conspirators were members of Payne Memorial A.M.E. Church, my parents' chosen place of worship. The plot was engineered by Miss Tread's sister-in-law, Ada Treadwell, who was extremely envious of my parents, and obsessively covetous of my mother's friendship with Miss Tread.

Although an involuntary witness to this *film noir,* I could not comprehend at the time or empathize with Sandra's anguish, terror, and despondency. For, in this moment she lost the respect and admiration of her father, her knight in shining armor.

Sandra was born July 22, 1947. My father was released from the Army the prior year. Overlaying the trauma he witnessed and survived during World War II with the notion of intimacy surely would have represented a significant emotional shift for him. Mom's grandfather was terminally ill, a victim of mesothelioma contracted during his decades of working in the coal mines. It was during the period in which Mom was preoccupied with helping Granny care for Grandpa Franklin that Sandra was born. Her birth heralded Dad's quest to reset the arc of his career path as he began his dental studies at the University of Iowa in Iowa City.

Sandra was Dad's little princess. Although she behaved as such as long as he was around, in his absence a power struggle with my mother would play out as Sandra threw tantrums and tried all sorts of stunts. For her part, Mom was intent upon teaching Sandra that her id was not as durable as Mom's iron will. Among the many tales Mom shared on this theme, one stands out from all the others.

On a cold winter's day, Sandra, a toddler, sat in the back seat as Mom struggled to master the manual transmission of their Model-A Ford on the icy hills of Iowa City. Mom had placed Sandra in the back seat beside Mom's sizable handbag with explicit instructions not to stand up. I think this was around 1950; there would have been no seatbelts. It was not uncommon to see traffic cops at busy intersections in town, directing traffic. As Mom drove, Sandra ignored her warnings about standing up in the back seat, and several times stood to peer out of the back window. Traffic was somewhat heavy, and the roads were slick with snow and melting ice. As Mom inched up a hill in the middle of town, a traffic cop, standing in the intersection, threw up his hand suddenly to halt her progress. Mom was terrified. She struggled to negotiate the steep incline without slipping backwards, accelerating just enough to regain forward traction. All the while, Sandra was out of her seat again as the lurching car caused her to lose her balance and fall onto the floor. The traffic cop beckoned Mom forward, as Sandra grabbed the handles of Mom's handbag in her chubby little fingers, climbed back into the seat, and with all her might, swung the handbag at Mom's head. Observing the incident, the traffic cop stopped the flow of all traffic initially to assess Mom's ability to hold the car steady and not crash. However, this public safety response quickly devolved into a scene straight out of *I Love Lucy*. Recovering from the shock, Mom secured the Model-A's on the incline, snatched Sandra from the backseat, still firmly clutching the handbag. Mom pinned her down on her lap, pulled up the layers of petticoats, and proceeded to spank her bottom with the purse, all the while admonishing the toddler with each strike, "I … told … you … not … to … stand up in the seat! And don't you … *EVER* … hit … me … like … that … if you … want to … see … tomorrow!" The traffic cop was laughing uncontrollably while holding up traffic as his eyes met Mom's. Mortified – by the calamity she could have caused by her novice shifting abilities – Mom slammed into first gear, and with the precision of a NASCAR driver accelerated forward, steering the Model-A through the intersection and onto level ground. This incident was a template for the constant power struggle between Sandra and Mom, lasting well into Sandra's teenage years.

At age 15, on this horrific night, Sandra saw her safety zone evaporate – perhaps forever – as Dad, her knight in shining armor, tried to come to her aid as he struggled on the floor with Mr. Tread. She let him down. She destroyed a piece of his soul. And it was doubtful the breach in their special bond would ever be repaired. Indeed, it was this bond she cherished so desperately, which motivated the incessant competition with Mom for Dad's affection.

Sandra's baby girl was adopted anonymously at birth. Prior to her delivery, all paperwork was completed and registered with the court allowing the adopting couple to claim the baby. It is unlikely that Sandra was allowed to see or hold her newborn. She remained in Des Moines for the next three years, finishing high school and enrolling in the local college. Eventually she was allowed to return home, and transferred to the University of Northern Iowa in Cedar Falls, just seven miles from Waterloo.

For a time, things seemed relatively normal. But one fateful Saturday afternoon while my sister and I were visiting with Miss Tread, Ada Treadwell knocked at the back door and came inside to join in the conversation. Ada was in high spirits. She spoke to Miss Tread and expressed surprise that Sandra was present. She grabbed my sister by the hand as though they were best friends, saying she would like to introduce Sandra to someone visiting her home. "It will only take a moment," Ada said, "I caught a ride with them over here, but they'll be leaving directly." Sandra followed Ada out to a parked car. I trailed behind, but could not see into the car. I remember my sister leaning in to speak to someone in the back seat. When she turned away from the car, Sandra looked as if she had seen a ghost.

What my sister saw was a couple in the backseat holding up a child they had adopted. As Ada explained, the child they held was Sandra's own. Looking back, this experience could have been Sandra's undoing. She did not tell our parents or Miss Tread about this incident until she confessed she was pregnant again by the same vagrant, six months later. The shock of seeing her firstborn so unexpectedly drove her to seek this guy in desperation, hoping he would help her reclaim their "love child."

The prevailing myths[1] about unwed mothers during the 1950's and 1960's held:

---

[1] Ann Fessler, *The Girls Who Went Away: The Hidden History of Women Who Surrendered Children for Adoption in the Decades Before Roe v. Wade* (New York: Penguin Group, 2006), 29-54.

babies surrendered for adoption were willingly and eagerly given up; the surrendering mothers suffered no sense of loss; and, of course, anyone who got pregnant was a slut. On the contrary, these marginalized, unwed mothers suffered real trauma, feeling an ongoing sense of worry about their surrendered children – a feeling some studies have equated with having a loved one who is *missing in action*. It is the idea that her child is alive, out there in the world somewhere, so will she run into him or her on the street one day? Furthermore, these women were told by every authority figure in their lives, "Don't ever tell anyone because people will think less of you. No man will ever want to marry you if he knows you were such a bad, slutty girl." But the majority of the women processed through homes for unwed mothers got pregnant from their very first sexual encounter – not because they were slutty, but because they were naïve.

At the same time, the prevailing sexual hypocrisy of the period placed no such blame, negative labels, or responsibility on male counterparts in these scenarios. The males went unscathed or were heralded as Casanovas.

It was only with the emergence of the Women's Movement in the 1970's that these maternity-home victims begin to wrestle with the realization that they had been duped.

Back to my family. Learning of Sandra's second pregnancy by the same vagrant, my parents realized they must send her away again. Their hopes were dashed that she would ever fulfill her incredible potential. They doubted they could ever reconnect with their daughter. This time they arranged for her to move to Minneapolis and live with Audrey and Linton Scott. Audrey was a distant cousin to Willa Mae and like Willa Mae, she attended Mom's Sunday school class so many years earlier. Linton Scott was a minister and student of theology from Jamaica. Rev. Scott was (and remains to this day) committed to outreach among underserved boys. He and his wife were very close to my parents. Mom and Dad had a great deal of respect and confidence in this young couple. Sandra would live with the Scotts until her salary from the Minneapolis Federal Reserve Bank enabled her to lease her own apartment, several years later.

When Sandra was a child, an innocent romp in the grass could lead to hives and debilitating fits of wheezing, sometimes severe enough to require hospitalization. Not only was she allergic to grass, but also to the rich soil in which it grew. Mom found it necessary to limit Sandra's play areas to indoor spaces, which severely restricted her interaction with the neighborhood children. Perhaps this isolation hindered her emotional and social development. From the time she entered kindergarten her curiosity and all-consuming drive to gain her peers' acceptance presaged, no doubt, her painful adolescence.

Perhaps this explains my sister's willingness to place her confidence in the least deserving people—people like Ada, whom Sandra should have known was jealous and envious of our parents' position in the community. Although these circumstances were tragic, they failed to harm my father's reputation as Ada and others from our church family intended. Nevertheless, when Dad announced to Mom that he was "leaving this Godforsaken state", I imagine his grievances extended beyond being denied surgical privileges at the town's hospitals. Our family's epic betrayal by fellow church members could not have been far from his mind.

From the age of four Sandra displayed an uncanny photographic memory. She could recall anything she heard, read, or saw with amazing accuracy—and the recall was lasting. She had the ability to remember an image with such stunning clarity and detail that it was as though the image remained in view. This was particularly true with numbers and music. Seeing her aptitude Mom sat Sandra on the piano bench and taught her to play. Sandra displayed such an incredible gift and affinity for music, Mom hoped music could counterbalance the privation of being unable to play freely outside. My parents sought the best teachers available, and eventually found an enigmatic piano and organ instructor, Margaret Dravis. Margaret had been accepted as a student at Juilliard in 1928. However, the stock market crash in '29 decimated her father's real estate holdings, and dashed her hope of studying in New York. She remained in Waterloo to assume management of the apartment buildings the family was able to retain. Eventually she assumed ownership of the properties, augmenting her income by teaching piano and scoring music for regional bands. Margaret possessed perfect pitch and the ability to hear instrumentation in her head, which she transferred to paper as easily as one might drink a glass of water. Despite the plebeian Waterloo of the 1950's, Margaret Dravis schooled Sandra in advanced music theory, harmony, and piano pedagogy, which she absorbed like a sponge. She coached Sandra in the distinct form, fit, and function of fingering techniques, the bio-physics of controlling pressure points at one's fingertips. She taught Sandra how to invoke gradations of volume and tone from the instrument. Still, around her peers Sandra hid her musical and academic talents as best she could, hoping to blend in. This behavior became another serious point of contention between Sandra and her mother.

Sandra's life was a profusion of remarkable contradictions. Her actions and attitudes were often driven by extreme empathy for others. She was completely unable to discern correctly a person's character, preferring, I suppose, to believe in some universal goodness that seldom materialized. For example, Sandra was generally unable to follow sinister plots in movies and television dramas. She expressed confusion and utter surprise when the story line revealed an obvious villain had perpetrated some sinister misfortune. We found it necessary to explain the twists and turns in the story, which she misinterpreted or missed altogether. This deficit rendered her forever vulnerable to the manipulation and humiliation of her classmates, but their abuse only strengthened her resolve to win their acceptance.

During her college years Sandra was less shy about her talent, and discovered she possessed the technical facility of a concert pianist. Her emotionally driven personality imbued her performances with uncanny artistic expression as well. Her musical prowess included both the piano and the pipe organ. Amazingly, she could read any piece of music once and master its form and composition. She practiced to perfect her technique with particularly difficult passages, but she could recall the entire work at will, even after months or years of not performing the piece. Perhaps for her, music was little more than an escape from the realities of her world, but for decades I found it incomprehensible that she did not parlay her incredible gifts into a career.

By 1970 it seemed Sandra had found her footing in Minneapolis. The Scott family proved to be a safe haven for her as she even began recording "live" piano soundtracks for Rev. Scott's weekly evangelist radio broadcasts. She found steady employment, and contemplated pursuing her music degree at the University of Minnesota. During this time, she somehow fell into the company of an aspiring attorney, LaJune Thomas, who heralded from a social background very similar to ours. Sandra seemed to open up with LaJune as they shared the excitement and anticipation of launching their respective careers.

I believe it was this new-found optimism that prompted Sandra to find an efficiency apartment on the perimeter of Loring Park near downtown Minneapolis. The location afforded her the luxury of walking to work. One day as she walked home after work, she found herself captivated by *Beethoven's Piano Sonata No. 8* drifting from the open window of a brownstone walk-up. She paused under that window with her eyes closed, imagining herself at the keyboard. Suddenly the sonata was interrupted by terse instructions from a demonstrative female voice, correcting some technique critical to the character of the music. Intrigued, and led by her go-where-angels-fear-to-tread id, she entered the building, discovering she had happened upon a piano studio. As she stood listening in the hallway, a stern older woman suddenly confronted her about her loitering. Sandra shocked the stranger by commenting on the passage of the sonata in such a descriptive manner the dowager instantly recognized her to be a very serious piano student. The woman invited her into the studio as the student's session was concluding, and following a polite verbal exchange, invited Sandra to play. Sandra seated herself at the piano and commenced her own distinctive interpretation of *Beethoven's Piano Sonata No. 8*, the trigger that initially drew her attention to this obscure brownstone. The dowager, we discovered, was a retired concert pianist of considerable international repute. She accepted Sandra as an acolyte and they became a formidable team over the next year, concluding with Sandra's victory as the grand champion of a notable piano competition akin to the Van Cliburn International Piano Competition in Fort Worth, Texas.

So it was that in the winter of 1972 – my junior year in high school – Mom, Dad, and I piled into our 1969 Pontiac Bonneville Brougham and made the 4-hour trek to Minneapolis. Our ultimate destination was the Northrop Memorial Auditorium on the University of Minnesota's Minneapolis campus where we witnessed Sandra take the stage with the Minnesota Symphony to perform *Tchaikovsky Piano Concerto No. 1 in B Flat Minor*. This was a triumphant moment for Mom, who had envisioned Sandra, not necessarily embracing the rigors of touring as a concert pianist, but at least established as a recording artist for *Deutsche Grammophon* or *RCA Red Seal Records*. It was surreal to have this stolen moment watching Sandra take command of the Steinway concert grand accompanied by the Minnesota Symphony before a sold-out auditorium. This was Sandra – not in our living room or in church – this was Sandra publicly and effortlessly displaying her unique artistry and mastery of this instrument. I vividly recall watching my mom clutch the breast of her black lamb evening coat. As the audience burst into applause, tears streamed down Mom's cheeks. Dad sat tall, and applauded proudly. Sandra rose from the Steinway to a rambunctious standing ovation, and shook the hand of the conductor, Stanislaw Skrowaczewski. I looked at my sister standing regally in that turquois blue velvet strapless gown surrounded by a 90-piece symphony clad in black tuxedos and satin gowns. I thought, *Who is this person? Is she really a part of our family? Am I truly related to her? Where has she been all of my life? I'm seventeen and I am cheering for a familiar stranger – why is that so?*

Although we all were elated, it is possible that Sandra was apprehensive about the prospect of breaking through the bullet-proof glass preventing black women from joining the ranks of concert pianists. Yes, it was the 1970's but just two decades before, Nina Simone (aka: Eunice Kathleen Waymon) – a piano virtuoso – was shut out of the prestigious Curtis Institute of Music in Philadelphia, despite a well-received audition. Nine days before her death in 2003, the Curtis Institute of Music awarded her an honorary degree. Likewise, Roberta Flack (a child prodigy who so excelled at classical piano that Howard University awarded her a full music scholarship) was also shut out of the classical piano world. Both these phenomenal women went on to forge iconic musical careers, but neither was supported in her original pursuit: conquering the world stage as black female concert pianists.

In addition to the opportunity to debut with the Minnesota Symphony, another benefit of winning that piano competition was an audition with André Watts, who was booked as a featured artist for Minnesota Symphony season ticket holders that season. Watts was "discovered" in the mid-sixties by Leonard Bernstein. By the early seventies he gave 150 performances per season with bookings confirmed three years in advance. Winter seized Minneapolis the day of the audition, but Sandra went to work at the Federal Reserve Bank as usual, and arranged to meet her old friend, Audrey Scott, at Northrop Memorial Auditorium that evening. Audrey warned Sandra that she may arrive a few minutes late, but to not wait for her. Early that afternoon, however, Audrey received a call from daughter's school, informing her of a debilitating asthma attack that sent the child to the emergency room for treatment. Audrey went to the hospital, and remained at her daughter's side until the child was released. It was after 10 p.m. when Audrey finally made it home through the winter storm. As soon as she put her daughter to bed, Audrey called Sandra eager to hear the juicy details of the audition. Sandra answered the phone to a barrage of questions: "Was Watts as handsome as he appeared to be on TV? What was he like? What did he say?" Audrey paused, waiting for Sandra to respond, but there was only silence. With Audrey's persistent prodding, Sandra confessed she did not audition. She showed up at Northrop Auditorium, but waited outside the concert hall for Audrey while her audition slot came and went. Not seeing Audrey, Sandra caught a bus and went home. Audrey nearly went into shock, apologizing and explaining she had been at the hospital emergency room with her daughter. She implored, "Why didn't you just go inside and play?" Sandra said simply that since her friend did not show up she felt she should just go home. None of this made any sense, and for years Audrey felt unduly responsible for Sandra's retreat from a once-in-a-lifetime opportunity. But that was Sandra.

Although she tested at a genius level IQ (somewhere north of 170), and excelled at just about anything she attempted, Sandra failed to maintain steady employment. Whenever she was offered a promotion she simply stopped showing up for work, choosing instead to fade into the shadows. Looking at this today with fresh eyes, I can attribute this flight reflex to the trauma (which I referred to earlier) of having been a teenage unwed mother.

While interning at General Mills' James Ford Bell Technical Center in the summer of 1973, I lived with my sister in her efficiency apartment. In the fall I would begin my studies in chemical engineering at The University of Iowa in Iowa City, but for the summer I was free to embark upon an adventure with this enigmatic figure – my big sister. I was genuinely excited to establish a bond with my only sibling. She was delightful, and seemed equally excited to welcome me into her home. I grew up practically as an only child, as Sandra was sent away eleven years earlier. I wonder now why we never talked about her trauma? And why I was estranged from my one and only sibling?

She had a myriad of wonders to show me as she introduced me to her adopted home city, which was being transformed at the time by multiple urban renewal projects. Minneapolis was a city of nearly 500,000, while the Minneapolis–St. Paull metropolitan area was home to nearly 2.5 million in the 1970's. My senses were on overload by the sheer scale of the metropolis, which dwarfed Waterloo. I was in the Land of Oz, and my anchor was this amiable stranger.

Sandra was employed at the Minneapolis Federal Reserve Bank. Her department counted worn currency scheduled to be destroyed and replaced. Her eidetic ability became suspect when she quickly caught an erroneous transaction receipt as it passed her workstation on its way to be translated into punch cards for computer processing. The tally on the receipt did not agree with the amount of currency attributed to that particular financial institution. She suddenly jumped up from her station and ran up several flights of stairs to intercept the incorrect punch cards before they could be processed. Her actions saved the bank millions and for her efforts she was followed for four weeks by the FBI, to and from work, and around downtown Minneapolis. She arrived home one day, paranoid that she was being followed, which no one believed because she was so "ditzy" about peoples' actions and intentions. However, a few days later she was approached at the bank by agents of the FBI who admitted they had been trailing her to determine whether she represented a threat. Of course, Sandra did not have a threatening bone in her body.

In the wake of her triumphant performance with the Minnesota Symphony, Sandra garnered the attention and respect of professional keyboard musicians in and around the Twin Cities area. To supplement her income– and just for fun – Sandra landed a second job as the assistant organist for the Hennepin Avenue Methodist Episcopal Church. This was easy money. She only had to attend choir rehearsals on

Wednesday or Thursday evenings, be on call for Sunday services, and play the occasional wedding or funeral as needed. Besides, the church was only a three block walk from her apartment. Others were astonished that she could walk in and win instant approval from this major institution. After all, the Church was an impressive operation with an annual budget approaching $15 million and a congregation of several thousand. But my sister fit comfortably into the operation. Her amiable personality quickly positioned her as one of the "daughters" of the church – at least that's how members of the chancel choir regarded her. One such couple, Dr. and Mrs. James Haun adopted Sandra as one of their daughters. Both sang in the chancel choir. My internship with General Mills could be attributed to Sandra's friendship with the Hauns. Dr. Haun was Senior Vice President of Engineering at General Mills. Although I did not enjoy any personal favors, I always knew Dr. Haun kept me under his watchful eye. I debated with him whether to transfer to Texas A & M or the University of Texas at Austin when my family moved to Dallas in 1974. On his recommendation, I selected the University of Texas.

The summer of 1973 with my sister proved to be quite enjoyable. I found her to be bubbly and adventuresome. Although brilliant, she was a terrible housekeeper, so the task of keeping the tiny efficiency apartment livable fell to me. Yet I recall weekly treats of White Castle® mini burgers on the nights following her choir rehearsal gig. Saturday's were pizza night. We ordered in and watched film noir on her tiny black and white portable TV. Once a month she would scrounge tickets to some event and we would go together as giddy schoolchildren. That's how I came to spend an evening at the Guthrie Theater, basking in the serenades of the incredible Sarah Vaughn.

Weekdays, I was absorbed in my projects at General Mills, but on the weekends I set out to explore the evolving downtown areas of Minneapolis. Returning to that Loring Park efficiency one Saturday afternoon, I was introduced by Sandra to Frank, a ruggedly handsome and stocky Scotsman. Frank was an ex-special forces operative who survived his deployment to Vietnam and now worked as a fireman for the Hennepin County Fire Department. He seemed very comfortable, and excited to spend time with my sister. He treated me in the manner I remembered from my days rolling on the front lawn as a five-year-old with Charlie Hill – seemingly a lifetime ago. Frank always displayed a Jimmy Stewart-like chivalry when he was with Sandra, carrying her books or packages, holding doors open for her, escorting her arm-in-arm as they walked. He was particularly excited that she took an interest in his projects renovating small apartment buildings with his buddies from the firehouse. I was enamored by this gentle giant, and very happy that he treated her with the respect and genteel care never afforded her in Waterloo. Frank wanted to marry Sandra. He wanted to get engaged and meet our parents, but she seemed to politely ignore his persistent though respectful pursuits. I don't recall what happened with Sandra and Frank, but when I returned for my summer internship the following year, sadly, he was no longer in the picture. She never spoke of him again.

One weekend during the fall of 1973 Sandra came home to Waterloo for a visit. While there, she attended a fundraising event at our parents' church. The elderly ladies responsible for counting the proceeds had not seen Sandra in several years, and she was full of stories to share. As she volunteered to assist them in auditing the proceeds, I stayed behind to provide her transportation home. At one point the ladies scolded Sandra for talking so much that she was distracting them from finishing the count. However, to the shock of all present, Sandra gleefully announced the tally at the end of the evening. The ladies questioned how she could possibly know the tally given that she had been talking rather than counting the money. Sandra innocently pointed to stacks of bills she had arranged on the table in discrete denominations. She quoted the tally of each stack, and the grand total. Whereupon several ladies spent the next half hour recounting the money, and to everyone's surprise Sandra's tally was correct. Astonished, the ladies asked how she was able to do this. Sandra explained that just like a card player shuffles a fresh deck of cards, she separated the denominations, hard-packed each stack of bills, and shuffled them. As the bills fluttered through her fingers she could count how many bills were in each stack, just like those electronic counting machines at a casino. Knowing how many bills were in each stack, she simply multiplied the number of bills by the respective denomination and provide a correct tally, all while telling her stories. I simply hung my head and chuckled, remembering the FBI agents.

When I returned to Minneapolis for my second summer internship, I met Sandra's girlfriend, LaJune Thomas. The two spent evenings and weekends window-shopping, attending various professional social events, and genuinely sharing girl time. It was heartwarming to learn that perhaps Sandra had finally found people who appreciated her for the wonderful and gifted person she was afraid to reveal in her hometown. LaJune was completing her degree in psychology at Augsburg College, and hoped to pursue a law degree at the University of Minnesota. I believe it was LaJune who floated the scenario of Sandra joining her at the University of Minnesota, saying how much fun it would be for the two of them to share their collegiate experience. LaJune's family was on par socially with our family. She had one brother whose first name I cannot recall so I will just refer to him as Mr. Thomas. I always believed LaJune empathized with the Sandra's silent struggles with Mom. Encouraged by the stylish LaJune, Sandra shed her frumpy clothes in 1974 for raiment that accentuated her statuesque physique. Upon my return to Minneapolis that summer, I saw a different Sandra. She seemed to have shed her protective shell. Just months before my return, Sandra walked through the doors of the School of Music at the University of Minnesota (unannounced and unscheduled) and asked to audition for a slot as a student of organ pedagogy. Miraculously she was not turned away, and without fanfare she mounted the Van Daalen organ – a two-manual, mechanical-action organ comprising 32 speaking stops and 41 ranks of pipes – and flawlessly performed Johan Sebastian Bach's *Taccata and Fugue in D Minor*. After her performance, Sandra was approached by the department chair, Dr. Heinrich Fleischer[2]. Dr. Fleischer was also a world-renowned scholar on the organ compositions of Johan Sebastian Bach, and was a visiting organ coach at Juilliard in New York. Although he did not accept undergraduate students, this renowned pedagogue invited Sandra to study under his tutelage. She accepted. There being no challenges to his decision, Sandra became Dr. Fleischer's sole undergraduate student. It is possible she did not fully appreciate this momentous opportunity.

When I returned to Minneapolis that summer, I learned Sandra had left the Federal Reserve Bank and was now employed with Chubb Insurance Company, performing legal transcriptions in their word processing pool. She was particularly suited to this task due to her photographic memory and amazing typing speed, exceeding 100 words per minute with a 99% accuracy rate. Her uncanny recall allowed her to create and populate spreadsheets in her head, and then produce the results as effortlessly as a macro-enabled Excel spreadsheet utility would do today. She retained her second job as assistant organist at the Hennepin Avenue Methodist Episcopal Church.

Midsummer, Sandra returned from one of her sessions with Dr. Fleischer as hot as a hornets nest. I asked what was wrong as she fumed with disgust. Her frustration was that Fleischer had never assigned her an entire composition to master and prepare for public performance. Instead, she complained, he assigned her specific passages from three or four composers to prepare for each lesson. She would spend three or four hours practicing at the church, not returning home until after

---

[2] Heinrich Fleischer (1912 – 2006) was an organist and pedagogue from Leipzig, Germany. Fleischer was a scholar of the late romantic style of organ playing, having completed in 1934 a PhD in musicology for organists from the Leipzig Conservatory, the finest school in Germany. "Heinrich Fleischer", accessed September 15, 2016, https://en.wikipedia.org/wiki/Heinrich_Fleischer.

10 or 11 p.m. The next day she would report for her lesson and on command execute the assigned passages. I burst into laughter because I had witnessed her running up the block to the church after supper to practice the night before the next day's lesson. Fleischer offered few corrections during those lessons, but would assign her a different series of discrete passages from the organ literature (e.g., *Couperin, Dubois, Saint-Saëns, César Frank, etc.*). Several weeks later Sandra returned home quite somber following a session with Fleischer. Again I inquired about the reason behind her mood. She told me that Fleisher had fired her as a student. Although she had been frustrated with him, she had bonded with his challenging demeanor. This sudden dismissal shook her very foundation. "When I challenged him," she recounted, "he told me I had been pulling the wool over his eyes for months. He explained the reason he had been assigning me these disparate passages was that he had been assessing the extent of my ability." She went on to relay that Fleisher told her his doctoral students had taken months to master the technical challenges of these same passages that she dashed off each week with very little difficulty. He told her that he suspected she had not been practicing on a daily basis, but that she was preparing just in time for her weekly lesson. His conclusion from his experiment to determine at what level he could identify her limits: There was little more he could teach her, and his commitments would no longer allow him to take attention away from his doctoral charges.

Over the next year Sandra changed her music major several times, finally settling on the emerging field of music therapy. She did not complete her undergraduate degree. Either she lost interest or the sudden brain aneurysm and the months of recovery broke the momentum of her collegiate studies. I continued my engineering studies at the University of Iowa, the family relocated to Dallas Texas, and I transferred to the University of Texas at Austin. Sandra continued her role as assistant organist at Hennepin Avenue Methodist Episcopal Church, and developed quite a reputation for her musicianship and congenial spirit among the congregation and the pastoral leadership. Easter Sunday in 1976 Sandra played the Sunrise Service, as well as the 11 o'clock service in which she was joined by a chamber orchestra (comprised of Minnesota Symphony members). The church catered an Easter brunch on the premises following the 11 o'clock services. Dr. and Mrs. Haun invited Sandra to sit at their table. As it happened, Sandra was seated across from one of the Twin Cities' most notable neurosurgeons. Halfway through the meal the doctor observed a sudden change in Sandra's posture. He ran over to catch her, bracing her by the shoulders as he shouted instructions immediately to call an ambulance. All the while he eased Sandra to the floor, cradling her neck and shoulders. She was having a grand mal seizure, and his embrace was intended to stem the damage. Sandra was rushed to the hospital where the same doctor was in charge of neurology. She had suffered a brain aneurysm caused by rupture in a cluster of malformed blood vessels. Her olfactory nerve was severed during surgery to control the bleeding and remove the malformed blood vessels. After hours of surgery, she was placed in the intensive care unit where she remained for a week. Although the prognosis was excellent, she lost her sense of smell. Once out of intensive care, Sandra remained hospitalized for a couple of weeks. Our parents consulted with her doctor to arrange her transfer to the care of a Dallas-based colleague of his. Sandra recovered at our parents' home, returning to Minneapolis after several months.

In 1984 Sandra left Minneapolis and moved to Dallas at the behest of our parents who maintained it would be safer for her to live closer to her family. I was consumed by my career, and did not pay much attention to my parents' machinations. I had not contemplated how close Sandra had come to dying in 1976. Still, her decision to come to Dallas brought me great joy. I invited her to live with me while she became acclimated to her new city. I was able to arrange for her to begin work in the quality assurance (QA) department of the defense contracting firm where I was employed. She was part of the documentation pool, responsible for publishing the myriad of technical and product specifications required by the U.S. Department of Defense (DoD). I taught my sister to drive a car and mentored her through her driving test and licensing. All seemed well for six months or so when she had a nervous breakdown at work, quoting scripture while sitting Indian-style on the floor outside the QA offices. She was assigned to Greenleaf Behavioral Health Hospital, a psychiatric facility, where she resided for the next three months (until her health insurance benefits were exhausted).

My parents and I rented and furnished an apartment for Sandra, prepaid three months' rent and funded the deposits for all utility services in time for her to move in after being released from Greenleaf. Sandra was allowed to return to her job at the defense contracting firm.

In 1986, Sandra was hired by the Dallas district offices of the Internal Revenue Service as administrative assistant to a rising-star executive. The staff, and particularly her boss, a young black female attorney, were astonished by her skills and ability to assimilate complex financial profiles into the barrage of investigative and analytical reporting that was required. This time her employment was interrupted when Sandra was arrested at the IRS offices and charged with writing hot checks at a 7-Eleven store one block from her apartment. We were all stunned. There was no logical reason for this. And why only at that 7-Eleven? Sandra's case went quickly to trial, and her boss was a character witness. The judge stated during his summation that despite the facts of the case, his assessment of Sandra's personality and demeanor indicated that she would not survive incarceration. He sentenced her to time served with three years' probation. To our complete amazement, the IRS allowed Sandra to return to work – her boss was delighted to have her back. Sandra's performance continued to astonish everyone. Her work was instrumental in garnering a major promotion for her boss to a Hawaii assignment. Unbeknownst to Sandra, her boss made Sandra's promotion and assignment to that same Hawaii post a condition of accepting the job. Her demand was approved and she eagerly shared the great news with Sandra. Offering her polite appreciation, Sandra left for the day, and never returned to those IRS offices again. But that was her way.

***

In 1987 Dad decided it was time to close his dental practice and retire. By then, Mom was a diabetes patient, and he was diagnosed with Alzheimer's. Having worked more than 55 years, he found the idea of retirement to be a challenge. He really did not know how to engage in hobbies or pursue an encore career. As Mom's health failed, I knew one of them would not remain on this side of the grass for very long after losing the other.

Sandra moved in with our parents, taking on the arduous role of a live-in caregiver. She was very effective at managing their health regimens, but I always carried suspicions that there was a self-serving, codependent aspect to her caregiving. My suspicions were fueled by her lackluster response to my numerous attempts to help her establish for herself an independent living arrangement. Fearing I may be too harsh on Sandra after their deaths, our parents named Sandra the executrix of their estate.

Mom succumbed to respiratory pulmonary failure 10 years later on May 1, 1997. Dad was completely silent at Mom's funeral. Sitting next to him, I saw a tear fall. When the funeral director handed him the ceremonial "key" to her casket, he seemed to exhale. He had gone through her dying with her and it was as if he was able to let go. It was over. After Moms funeral, Dad sort of perked up. That mischievous and amiable facet of his personality emerged. He wanted to go to social events. I remember attending a formal charity affair with my sister and him. He cut quite a figure in his tux. At the table during the banquet, he was charming and animated, entertaining the entire table with his witty anecdotes. My sister and I looked at each other as if to ask, *Who is this man?*

On November 23, 1997—three weeks after the banquet (and six months after my mother's death)—my father ate dinner, sat down for his customary 30 minute nap before watching his favorite television show, *Gunsmoke*. He died quietly of a massive stroke.

Our parents' lifelong goal was to remain in their home until their deaths. With Sandra's help, I am happy to say their goal was achieved. When the time came, they relinquished their rich lives and moved on to the next chapter without resistance or drama or fear.

With both parents deceased, Sandra and I had several options for the homestead. We could pay off the meager mortgage. We could renovate the property and lease it. Or we could sell it. Not surprisingly, I found Sandra indecisive. To my complete dismay she failed to work with me to accomplish any of the options available to us. Exasperated, I surrendered within two years of our parents' deaths all financial and inheritance claims to my sister. The last conversation I had with Sandra was on my birthday in 1999. After wishing me a happy birthday, she told me she had been evicted from the homestead and had moved in with a retired lady in the Oak Cliff area of Dallas. Her new landlord was also a member the church where I found myself on the day of her funeral. My sister and I were estranged from that day forward – for the last ten years of her life.

Lost in my reflections I was suddenly brought back to the funeral proceedings by the voice of my Uncle Jack, offering reflections of his own on Sandra's life. Uncle Jack had always been a shady character, having alienated nearly all of our family members with his shenanigans. I had not seen or spoken to him since my Uncle Mac's funeral in 1992. He was now 84. I was shocked to see how lonely and forsaken he seemed. But then, the last person on earth he had not alienated was lying in the casket before him.

Sitting there, I thought once more about the summer of 1973 when I lived with my sister in Minneapolis. What if I had been able to talk with her intelligently about the trauma in her life? What if we had been able to discuss the depth and breadth of what we *both* experienced in 1962? In what wonderful ways might the past ten years have been different for us?

Suddenly the service was ending. The pallbearers methodically closed Sandra's casket in preparation for rolling it out of the sanctuary toward the waiting hearse. The sanctuary seemed to take on a synthetic, slightly stale odor. I struggled to make a gracious exit up the aisle behind my sister's coffin. I found it difficult to breathe. I needed fresh air as quickly as possible. As I reached the portico, I found it impossible to discern any logic from the din of deafening conversation occurring there. Getting away from those people was paramount. I caught a glimpse of Cousin Bettye, and as our eyes met, time seemed to stand still and simultaneously race backwards. Bettye and Sandra were childhood buddies and kept in contact throughout most of their lives. She was a year older than my sister, and nine years older than me. Although we were never close, it was Bettye who found me on Facebook, alerted me of my sister's passing, and kept me informed of my Uncle Jack's plans to choreograph this funeral. Sandra's burial would be in Waco near my father's siblings, but I had no desire to return to Waco for the graveside service. Instead I made plans to drive to Austin and spend a few days in quiet reflection. I had not seen Bettye since her father's funeral in 1992. She and her husband, Walter, moved back to Austin from Walter's home in Jamaica, Queens, New York only weeks before my sister's death. Anyway, I fled the funeral, crossing the parking lot in the direction of the car I arranged for the Austin escape. A dear friend gave me the keys to her showroom-new Cadillac CTS for the weekend, insisting that I surround myself with ultra-reliable comfort in my time of mourning. At the time I protested this kind but unnecessary gesture. My beater would get me there and back just fine. Fortunately, I lost the debate and reluctantly accepted the gesture on the faith that my friend was not known for irresponsible flights of fancy.

Through an invisible fog I found the vehicle, inserted myself in the sumptuous cocoon, and drove away.

I was numb. I don't recall much of the first 30 minutes of the drive. At some point the air around me cooled as I found myself wrestling with pangs of anger, relief, disappointment, and an eerie sense of abandonment. It was a fact – I was officially an orphan. Mom was gone. Dad was gone. Now Sandra had left me. Although my sister and I had been estranged, I was angry that she had left me without warning. Another 15 minutes passed as I struggled to find solace in the methodical low pitched whine of the tires spinning over the roadbed. My emotional discomfort eased itself in the uncanny contemplation that by all accounts, Sandra had been a consistently peaceful, and deeply spiritual thought leader in her church community. This was the parishioners' decade-long truth about the familiar stranger. How was this possible?

A few days later I contacted Bettye and Walter, arranging to spend an afternoon visiting them in their new home. This was a chance to catch up and fill in the past 17 years of our lives. Bettye shared that she often thought about my sister and her life struggles, wishing that she could have experienced more happiness in her life. She said, "I saw Sandra express true happiness a few years ago when she attended a family reunion in Brazoria County. She danced in among the extended family carrying an umbrella as a shield from the hot sun – and she was beaming! At one point she asked me, 'Am I being too happy?' I simply told her to enjoy herself." Bettye went on to describe a memory from Sandra's graveside service. "The casket was open and one curl of her hair was blowing gently in the fall breeze. I thought to myself, *She is finally at peace.*"

When I was four, my father used to sit me on the edge of the kitchen sink and wash my face with a sopping wet washcloth, which as I experienced it, was akin to waterboarding. He did not intend any harm, rather it was his perfunctory manner of dispatching the task of washing me up for some spur-of-the-moment destination. I never complained about it. I simply held my breath until the wet washcloth was removed, but the fear was there. I was never able to properly master the breaststroke because I could not breathe with water dripping across my face. It was many years before I finally conquered this phobia by forcing myself to place my face in front of the pelting showerhead, and breathe, to prove I would not drown.

The statutory rape of my sister was enough to convince me sex was a terrible weapon used to inflict infinite pain on unsuspecting people. Sex could hurt people and ruin their lives. Sex was to be feared and sexual arousal could be life-threatening. Subconsciously, I feared being perceived as a social predator. In truth, I did not interpret sexual desire in any normal or healthy context until I was nearly 30. In reality, there is no reason to fear a water-soaked towel covering your face. There is no reason to fear sexual arousal. Yet it amazes me how a single incident could produce a false assumption, and how profoundly such an assumption may affect one's attitudes and actions – for decades. If this is a credible example of my psychological scarring, then I can only imagine the trauma visited upon my sister's life as she lived through rape, two pregnancies, and then surrendered both babies at the end of nine months.

In Waterloo, we were the family on the hill, destined to be perennial outsiders, envied by most, hated by some, and loved by few. Ultimately, the wonder of the community of my early childhood years would be overshadowed by my perception of its true nature. Although I saw glimpses of truth during my high school years, only decades later could I begin to appreciate fully the depths of deception, ill will, and meanness my family endured there. We never sought family counseling for the emotional scarring we suffered, but I feel very strongly our entire family was violated. We were all victims of the statutory rape that occurred in 1962, and yet, it was Sandra who suffered most.

Following Sandra's death, I thought about the others – Granny, Miss Tread, Lizzie, Mom, and Dad – all deceased. I understand now that the strength I gleaned from these indelible characters paled in comparison to the hope imprinted by the familiar stranger – Sandra Louise Harvey – into my familial DNA. I believe it was hope that kept her going despite her trials, foibles, and tribulations. Hope brought her to a peaceful and productive place in her final decade. I could not anticipate that six years after her passing I would need to build upon my sister's hope to survive the greatest test I would ever face. Thank you, Sandra ... from the bottom of my heart!

PART II

8 Discovery Begins

Throughout my life I have enjoyed the luxury of frequent travel. These excursions began with my parents when I was just two years old with road trips to Anaheim, California for the wondrous and magical Disneyland experience. I remember riding the *Alice in Wonderland* "Mad Tea Party" spinning teacups, and losing my plastic sword down the throat of Tick-Tock the crocodile, made famous by the Disney animated movie, *Peter Pan*. Subsequent trips whisked me away to Niagara Falls, the Rocky Mountains, the Grand Teton and Yellowstone National Parks, the Pacific Northwest, Las Vegas, and the Grand Canyon.

When I was twelve I accompanied my parents on their 25th wedding anniversary to Hawaii. We spent three weeks there, visiting Oahu, Kona, and Maui. At that impressionable age, it was Maui that touched me deeply. I had never witnessed topography, surf, or sunsets as vivid as those of Maui. I think the experience exceeded the capacity of my preteen mind and spirit to comprehend. Living on the plains of Iowa, I did not know such exquisite and exotic beauty could be found in land or people. The experience left me afraid to return for fear that my memories were imagined, and seeing Maui again might destroy the beautiful imagery in my head.

I continued to travel frequently as I embarked on a career in chemical engineering with Dow Chemical USA, making customer care calls to remote locations in Utah, Montana and Northern California. Later, both employment and volunteer pursuits sent me globe-trotting through Great Britain, Germany, France, Spain, Austria, Switzerland, and the Yucatan. These places plus Montréal, Canada, and the San Francisco Bay Area captured my imagination, and each uniquely welcomed me as if I had been born there. New York, Chicago, San Diego, Washington DC, Boston and Miami were intriguing, but less so.

Despite my former travels, by 2015 I had become a vacation-challenged workaholic. My love affair with travel ended on September 11, 2001, when the world as we knew it, ceased to exist. I was enjoying a California vacation. I rented a Jaguar in San Francisco and spent a week meandering south towards San Diego through the spectacular scenery on the Pacific Coast Highway. As I reached my destination, my vacation was interrupted. I was dispatched to Irvine to meet Josh, a salesman from New Jersey, for a consult with a corporate client in Orange County. Exchanging the Jag for a car that could be expensed, I checked into a hotel near John Wayne Airport. After my meeting, I prepared to catch a flight home on the morning of September 11th. Standing in front of the mirror in my hotel room, brushing my teeth, I caught a glimpse on TV of the first World Trade Center tower as it fell. I assumed this was a new movie, and made no connection whatsoever between the images I saw, and my travel itinerary. I continued to get dressed. Not until I met Josh for breakfast did I discover that the TV images were real, and

America was apparently under attack. A phone call alerted me that my flight would be delayed, but a subsequent call informed me my flight had been cancelled. In time, not only were all airplanes grounded, but also the banks were closed and secured by the National Guard.

With no flight and only a little money, Josh and I found ourselves trapped in Orange County for four days. Stranded travelers filled hotel lobbies where free food and drinks were available while they lasted. On the fourth day Josh's bank opened. Now with sufficient funds, we checked out of the hotel, loaded our luggage in the trunk of the rental and made our way east on Interstate 10 through throngs of military vehicles and personnel. It was like a scene from *Mad Max: Beyond Thunderdome*, except Mel Gibson and Tina Turner were nowhere to be found in this director's cut. On the drive to Texas we stopped a couple of times to check into a hotel but only found more stranded travelers and a few rooms set aside for showers. Otherwise all rooms were booked. We kept driving. After about eight hours on the road (I believe we were in New Mexico), we came upon a three-mile stretch of highway where one National Guardsman was posted every six feet or so. The freeway was closed. We were routed off the interstate through a desert town of mostly mobile homes, as guardsmen with German Shepherds and Dobermans checked each car, apparently looking for arms and explosives. It took us nearly three hours to travel five miles. Things were pretty normal after that. By the time we made it to Dallas, the airport was open. I dropped Josh off at DFW and headed home. My condo never looked so good.

It took fourteen years, but in the spring of 2015 I decided it was time to get over my personal 9-11 saga. Having gathered the courage to return to Maui, I booked a flight for my 60th birthday and made reservations at the Westin Ka'anapoli Ocean Villas Resort in northern Maui. During the hour's drive from the airport to the resort along the western coastline I was hypnotized by the beauty and tranquility of the island and intoxicated by the fresh ocean breezes infused with jasmine and other floral scents. I could almost taste the air. In those first hours on the island my childhood experience was fully affirmed. I sent thanks to my parents in heaven for having given me the magical gift of Maui so many decades earlier.

However, my love affair with this enchanted place was horrifically interrupted by debilitating respiratory problems. Surrounded by exceptional and exquisite beauty, I found myself unable to walk more than 100 yards at a stretch. Breathing was not painful, but for some reason I could not take in sufficient air to sustain myself without frequent stops to rest for a minute or two. I attributed this sudden shortness of breath to physical exhaustion or possibly some unidentified allergy.

When I returned from my trip, I called my primary care physician (PCP), Dr. Washington, who had cared for my family since the mid-1980's. His specialty was internal medicine with a focus on stress-related health injuries and industrial workers compensation. Dr. Washington eschewed the inconvenience of insurance reimbursements, and required direct payment from his patients. He ordered a battery of diagnostic tests, including chest x-rays, EKGs, blood analyses, respiratory and stress tests, and sonograms of my lungs (totaling $4,000). But the tests yielded no conclusive results. In July Dr. Washington indicated during my appointment that he was reviewing my test results and would refer me to the appropriate specialist. Since my trip I had no recurrence of the shortness of breath, no pain or other physical symptoms, so there seemed to be no emergency. He assured me his office would be calling me for a consult within the next few weeks.

Near the end of July Dr. Washington's office called, but not with the information I expected. I was informed that he would soon be admitted to the hospital for surgery to relieve blood clots in his leg. At 65 he sported a trim physique that was the result of a rigorous fitness regimen followed religiously for 35 years. His office called me again a month later to alert me they would be scheduling my consult with Dr. Washington upon his return to his practice. But in early September he suddenly passed away. I was shocked to learn my friend of some 30 years had died. For decades I enjoyed the comfort and convenience of special access to my PCP. My shock was followed by my confusion and concern that my medical condition remained unaddressed. I struggled to think how I would find a comparable replacement within my health insurance network. After days of sifting through lists of physicians, I signed off of my online health plan and counseled myself to be quiet and think. In my experience, whenever I needed an expert to address a particular issue or problem, I had been able always to recall some connection – whether longstanding or fleeting – with the right person.

Several days of quiet contemplation passed before I remembered having dinner in April of that year with the wife of a colleague who was making plans to open a new family medicine practice. I remembered the conversation but it had not registered with me that she had practiced medicine for some 20 years. I simply knew her socially. When I checked my cell phone contacts and found her private cell number, I took it as a sign that I should probably reach out to her. I called Dr. Chowdhury, who was excited to invite me to have a conversation about her "concierge ultimate care" model. During my interview with her, I learned she had a lifelong passion to provide contextual medical and fitness support to her patients – a level of care that included relating a patient's age and health record with family medical history, as well as environmental factors and daily physical exertion. "Ultimate care" is also known as contextual medical fitness, the tenacious pursuit of intellectual certainty regarding the real-time impact of a patient's medical profile and lifestyle. Ultimate care does not rely solely on a prescribed punch list of tests, inoculations, annual physicals and routine diagnostics. Rather, this approach pushes beyond the boundaries of "that's good enough" to insulate a provider from medical malpractice, to a place where the patient's sustainable fitness and quality of life goals drive the doctor-patient relationship. No assumptions are made in an ultimate care scenario.

After my initial conversation with Dr. Chowdhury, I was convinced that she offered an improvement over the personal care I had received for decades from my late friend, Dr. Washington. So began a new journey to re-baseline my health profile and plan for the quality of life I desired as I entered my sixties. I told Dr. Chowdhury that maintaining mobility and vitality were my key objectives. I had already made adjustments to my nutrition and fitness regimen. We discussed options that were available to me through her concierge franchise partners that may shape a proactive approach to my future care. One of the first steps we agreed to was to focus on bringing my immunization profile in line with current standards. This involved some eight or nine booster inoculations to be administered over the next three months. On the Thursday before Christmas 2015, I visited Dr. Chowdhury's office to receive my pneumococcal pneumonia inoculation – the last in the series. She instructed her med tech to obtain a urine sample from me to round out my new medical baseline. The next day she called to alert me that unusual proteins were found in my urine. She suspected the cause to be bacterial and indicated she would attempt to grow a culture over the weekend. I informed her my two-week vacation would begin the following Monday.

The first day of my vacation, Dr. Chowdhury called to tell me that she was unsuccessful in growing a culture, which ruled out a bacterial infection. She was perplexed as to the source of the proteins and requested that I report to the emergency room at Baylor Scott and White Hospital to have the urinalysis rechecked. That is how I ended up spending the four days before Christmas in the hospital. It became a joke between Dr. Chowdhury and me that her tenacity stole Christmas, but saved my life.

Following Dr. Agha's instruction, I contacted Dr. Chowdhury the week after Christmas to let her know I needed an infectious disease specialist. She referred me to a colleague, Dr. Claire Brenner, and with her referral I was able to schedule an appointment with Dr. Brenner the week between Christmas and New Year's.

Weeks of analysis ensued between Dr. Brenner and Dr. Agha to determine the best course of action to save my life.

For the next six weeks I shared the details of my health crisis with no one but my manager at CVS Health, my place of employment. I had known JJ some 20 years from previous employment in the health services industry, and I was certain I could trust him with the evolving medical diagnosis.

When I saw Dr. Brenner, I learned the pathology results from Baylor (delayed, due to the skeleton staffing during the Christmas holiday) revealed my HIV and hepatitis B viral loads were shockingly low. The kidney biopsy proved the viral attack had persisted for at least 15 years. Left undiagnosed and untreated, my HIV viral load should have been in the millions, but in fact it was only slightly above 50,000. I was hospitalized for ten days in 1990 for a near-fatal food infection. Every year since then, I had been tested for viral infections. I questioned Dr. Brenner as to why my former PCP had not detected the HIV and hepatitis B infections. She explained it was impossible until recently to detect viral loads as low as mine with any degree of accuracy. Although today viral loads can be detected as low as 10, in years past a combination of testing and physical symptoms determined one's risk. Apparently, my immune system had kept my viral loads below the sensitivity of the available technology. Absent any discernible physical symptoms, I was cleared each year. I welcomed her explanation, and took solace that for 15 years my immune system *alone* had been effective In battling the viral infection.

The tests done at Baylor also showed I had been exposed to syphilis at some point in my life, but there was no way to tell immediately whether the virus was live, which would indicate recent exposure, or dead. To error on the side of caution, Dr. Brenner scheduled a six-week penicillin regimen to counter her suspicions that I may have also been exposed to syphilis. I learned that habitual drug users typically present a combination of HIV, hepatitis and syphilis – primarily through infected needles. Whenever one of these three infections is confirmed, the other two are likely to be present. I am not, nor have I ever been an intravenous drug user. I was absolutely sure there could be no live syphilis virus in my system, but I had no credibility at this point. I decided my best tact would be to cooperate and allow the tests they wanted so that they could obtain empirical evidence to support my claim.

The following Thursday at 11:30 a.m. I reported to Dr. Brenner's office to begin a series of penicillin injections. Two good-natured nurses led me into an exam room and requested that I pull down my tidy whities. At that moment I learned to set aside my personal pride and modesty. Next I was instructed to lean over the exam table with both arms stretched outward. Then, as in a game of rock-paper-scissors, one of the nurses would give the count, "One. Two. Three." and on cue each nurse simultaneously stabbed me in each butt cheek with her needle of penicillin. "Sir, you are going to feel a slight burn as the medicine is injected." I wanted to cry out to relieve the shock and awe of the experience. Instead, I took a quick, deep breath and remained silent until both needles were withdrawn. One of the nurses said happily, "All done." Over the next five weeks this routine would be repeated again and again. A couple of times one nurse would begin the count and the other nurse would say "Wait, I'm not ready." We would all chuckle, and the count would begin again. I would take a deep breath, and wait for the assault to end.

Further testing revealed a negative result: there was no live syphilis virus in my system. With this result I felt certain that my credibility as a patient was on the rise.

Much of January 2016 was a blur, obscured by my hectic work schedule as Advisor and Process Architect for the CVS Health Infrastructure Architecture Team within Enterprise Information Services (EIS). I received a phone call from JJ, my manager, during the first week of February. He asked if I were okay because he had audited several of my recent conference calls and noticed my verbal and written responses seemed slightly off. JJ indicated that he suspected no one else had noticed the change, and he attributed his recognition of the barely perceptible variation in my conduct to his long-time association with me. He suggested that I consider applying for short-term disability to allow time for my body to adjust to the antiviral therapy. JJ pointed out that since my hospitalization, I had been subjected to a significant amount of psychological trauma and physical duress related to the diagnosis of my renal failure. He went on to say it was his concern that, should I attempt to continue working, I was bound for a more serious breakdown. JJ's words hit me like an uppercut from a professional boxer. Was he saying he didn't want me on his team any longer? Was he just trying to cover his own ass? For the next few moments (which seemed like hours) I remained stunned by his comments. Then my subconscious mind locked onto his reference to our "long-time association."

JJ and I met when I enrolled in the accelerated executive educational track at LeTourneau University, a continuing education partner of Boeing Defense and Space (my place of employment at that time). The class was assembled for a special orientation session that evening in June 1994, and we were asked to break up into project teams. After about 20 minutes, people began to settle into groupings in each corner of the room, but I noticed one lone person sitting silently, hands clasped on his desktop. He was dressed in his policeman's uniform, complete with a loaded pistol, stun gun, and handcuffs attached to the patent leather belt. His polished shoes reflected their surroundings. I left my newly formed team, walked across the room and stood in front of him, extending my right hand, saying, "Hi, my name is Reggie, and I'd like you to be on my team." JJ rose from his seat and stood facing me. He was a few inches taller than I and his stance revealed a muscular frame that I would learn was the result of his many years of physical conditioning while in the Marine Corps. JJ should have been deployed in "Desert Storm", but suffered a back injury while repelling down the face of a mountain during a training exercise, just one week before his scheduled departure. After a medical discharge from the Marines he enrolled in a police academy and was now a licensed law enforcement officer in the DFW Metroplex. He looked at me sternly and shook my hand to accept my invitation. I led him across the room to my new team, saying "John (JJ) will be joining our team." To my surprise the team members each took an unwelcoming step backward. I responded to their body language saying, "He's on *my* team. You need to decide whether you will be, also!" We exchanged contact information, and that weekend he called me to ask, "You're not afraid of me? I don't intimidate you?" I remember chuckling as I responded, "You don't know my father. He's the most austere and intimidating person I have ever met. Therefore, I have no reason to feel threatened by you." That is how our lasting friendship began.

This memory passed before me in a few seconds, reassuring me his suggestion was made out of genuine concern for my wellbeing. I calmed down and told him I would contact human resources about a disability leave of absence. After speaking with HR, I agreed my last day of active duty would be Friday, February 12th. I notified JJ, and we both began preparations for my leave. He sought my temporary replacement while I prepared a briefing package containing the complete body of knowledge and information regarding my assignment. The following week I arranged to work from home, and hosted a midweek conference call with colleagues from Arizona, Rhode Island, and New Jersey. The call was scheduled for 11:00 a.m. I called in to the conference center and established the bridge. The purpose of the call to agree on the action plan critical for the project to move forward. However, it took 15 to 20 minutes to connect with everyone. There was a weather crisis developing on the East Coast and evacuations were underway at CVS Health facilities in Rhode Island and New Jersey. The East Coast colleagues joined the call from their mobile phones as they evacuated their offices and headed home. Nonetheless, the meeting proceeded, and the action plan was thoroughly reviewed. During the teleconference I received calls from Drs. Agha and Chowdhury at 11:45 a.m., which I could not answer or acknowledge for fear of compromising the active conference bridge. I knew the conference call would end shortly. My plan was to return both calls at that time.

When the conference call ended, I went to the kitchen for a drink of water, and then to my bedroom to rest for a few minutes before returning the missed calls. My few moments of peace and quiet were interrupted by obnoxiously loud banging on my neighbor's door (I thought). I continued to drink my water, but again I heard *BANG, BANG, BANG!* I looked out my bedroom window to find a large fire truck parked in front of my building with lights flashing. Only then did I realize my own front door – not my neighbor's – was being assaulted. I ran to the door and swung it open before the assailants could break it down, ready to give somebody a piece of my mind. In my haste I forgot that I was wearing only cotton briefs, and my hair was uncombed. My jaw dropped as I took in the visage of three larger-than-life firefighters poised to barge through my door. In a moment of panic I took several steps backwards.

I don't remember which one spoke to me but I heard, "Is Mr. Harvey here?"
"I'm he. What's going on?"
"Are you OK? You seem to be OK? Is there anything we can do for you?"
"Yeah, you can get away from my front door!" I was horrified to have these strangers see me nearly naked.
One of the firefighters continued, "We received a life emergency response request. Your doctors reported that your recent blood work indicated your phosphorus levels had risen to 7."
"What?"
"Your doctors were afraid your heart may have stopped. But you appear to be alright. You should be comforted to know that there are people who care about you enough to call for our assistance."

Was I dreaming? What just happened? I snapped back to reality while my floor shook as these oversized beasts stomped toward their fire truck. I slowly crossed the room to shut and lock my front door. As if in a trance I returned to my bed and picked up my cell phone. For a moment I could only stare at it, as I watched the fire truck depart. Then I suddenly burst into uncontrollable laughter, thinking about this scene that just played out. It really had not been a sketch from the *Carol Burnett Show* or *I Love Lucy* with me playing a leading role.

I dialed Dr. Chowdhury. She answered immediately, "Are you okay?" "Yes, I'm fine." I proceeded to recount the comedy that had played out in my living room moments earlier. As I was telling the story I realized the panic on the part of my doctors had been the genuine fear that I could have been dying.

Perhaps I had been in denial, but now I came face to face with the reality that my health was still indeed in a very fragile state.

9 A Little Help From My Friends

There is a significant difference between having a healthy self-interest and being selfish. I have championed this idea for a decade or more, but negotiating the survival of renal failure gives it new gravitas.

My initial appointment with the infectious disease specialist, Dr. Brenner, took place January 7, 2016. By then she had reviewed thoroughly the pathology reports from Baylor Scott and White Hospital. The abnormally low viral loads compared with the extensive damage to my kidneys led Dr. Brenner to recommend I begin a daily antiviral regimen consisting of three medications: Tivicay (50 MG, once daily/a.m.); Abacavir (300 MG, twice daily/a.m. & p.m.); and Epivir (5 ML, once daily/a.m.). She emphasized the importance of taking this cocktail consistently to effectively suppress the ability of the HIV and hepatitis B viruses to replicate themselves. Sustaining this antiviral therapy was a shared responsibility between Dr. Brenner and me. She would be responsible for reviewing, adjusting, and renewing the prescriptions, as well as monitoring the suppression of the viral loads. My responsibility was to get my prescriptions filled in a timely manner, and assure the drugs were always available. I had no idea how challenging it would prove to be to uphold my end of the bargain.

Dr. Brenner wanted me to start the antiviral therapy as soon as possible. So with prescriptions in hand, I visited my customary CVS retail pharmacy to acquire the drugs. I expected a 15-minute wait. My plan was to begin the therapy the next day. The pharmacy tech took the prescriptions to his computer station, keyed them into the prescription management support database, and asked whether there had been any changes to my prescription drug plan. I let him know there had been none. To my surprise he sighed heavily saying, "This is going to be a challenge. We have more problems with CVS pharmacy plans than with any third-party insurer." I assumed this comment was nothing more than sarcastic banter against a "rival" CVS business unit.

Ranked a Fortune 10 enterprise, in 2016 CVS Health was comprised of 51 independent health services businesses, employing nearly 250,000 people and generating over $153 billion in net revenues. One of the 51 health services business units is the CVS retail pharmacies, representing nearly 9600 stores in the United States. I am employed with Enterprise Information Services (EIS), which provides technology and digital communications capabilities to sustain the processing and daily delivery of nearly 2 million prescriptions. There had always been a measure of tension between CVS retail pharmacy operations and CVS EIS.

"We're going to have to submit your prescriptions to CVS Specialty Pharmacy (yet another of the 51 business units). Only Specialty Pharmacy is authorized to process and supply these particular drugs for you."

"You're joking, right?" I was under the impression my employment with CVS Health afforded me unfettered access to an extensive formulary through the CVS retail pharmacy system. I did not realize that the antiviral therapy components were managed outside the standard pharmaceutical formulary as *specialty drugs*.

"No, sir. You will have to contact Specialty Pharmacy directly to: establish an account with them; submit these prescriptions to their pharmacists for review and approval; make arrangements for any available copayment assistance; and schedule delivery of the drugs to either your home or a CVS Retail Pharmacy store location."

The 15-minute estimate exploded in my head like a Titan missile. As it was 5:30 p.m. when I presented the prescriptions, there was no way I was going to receive these drugs in time to begin therapy the next day. My angst diminished somewhat when I remembered CVS Specialty Pharmacy generated $250 million dollars in revenue per quarter. Obviously, it was a major operation and their processes would be well honed. Perhaps I would get the drugs in 2 to 3 days – not so bad, after all. *WRONG!* I spent the next seven days attempting to establish an account and submit the prescriptions. During the first few days I was routinely told that one or more of the prescriptions had not been received or recorded into my account profile. Arguments ensued over the ever-changing copayment for one of the drugs, ranging from $0 - $100 per month on any given day.

Towards the end of the week I went postal – so to speak – on a customer service agent. By then my rage had festered into a snarling crescendo. I nastily screamed into the phone, "Let's just cut the crap! We can stop playing this idiotic game, if you'll just admit *YOU'VE DECIDED TO KILL ME*, because it is evident that you people are *never* going to give me these drugs!" Did I really just say that? Did I? Oh shit! Had I used my *outside voice*? I continued, "*I need your help!* Every time I call it's a different story. Information that was retrieved 24 hours ago seems to magically disappear. I've been on the phone every day this week for 60 to 90 minutes per call trying to make arrangements for these drugs. I realize you are only working off of the information displayed on your terminal, and you don't control the information that is or is not properly retained in the system. I've been transferred to at least five of the 26 specialty pharmacy distribution centers, and with each transfer this conversation starts from scratch. I've been told 'you can't find the prescriptions', 'you don't have the drugs' at that facility, and 'there is no record of my insurance or co-pay assistance contracts'. *Do you people understand I am in renal failure and could die if I don't get these drugs?*"

In that moment I tried to make my situation *real* for the CVS customer service agent. My survival depended upon bringing the agent out from under her headset, through that phone and into my life. She had to understand there was a living, breathing human being attached to that conversation. My tirade was messy and unartfully articulated, but it was passionate, and the trepidation in my voice was authentic fear: I was afraid of dying. My outburst was fueled by raw emotion. The urgency of my tone transformed my "healthy self-interest" platitude into an urgent plea to save my life.

After an awkward silence I could hear the agent's fingers franticly typing as she informed me what could be done, and the sequence of events that should take place over the next several days. She encouraged me to call back and ask specifically for her should I have questions or further trepidation about the transaction. Before ending the call, she reviewed the details of my request with me to confirm that her record was complete.

This was my initiation into the role of medical advocate. I would find it necessary to negotiate the minefields of rules and regulations, insurance, access and delivery of health services. As a patient whose life hung precariously in the balance – subject to decisions made by people whom I would never meet – I could not sit back and wait to be rescued. I waged guerrilla warfare in a life-and-death struggle to encourage, cajole, and shame (when necessary) insurance providers, specialty pharmacy services, and human resource benefits specialists into acting in my best interest. The many moving parts of the healthcare system, I discovered, may not be counted on to deliver services as advertised in the slick and clever packaging. Nevertheless, underappreciated healthcare providers perform daily miracles, finding ways to provide care and life-saving treatment to patients despite often being handcuffed or blindfolded by the system in which they work. These men and women make it possible for a patient like me to cling to hope from day to day.

Despite my fragile health, I found it necessary to take steps to guarantee uninterrupted access to critical therapies as I waited my turn in the transplant queue. I marshaled all the skills attained through more than 40 years of professional employment to anticipate failures in case management protocols and processes. I leveraged my communication skills to encourage and inspire my medical team to do everything medically possible in support of my care and well-being. I certainly fumbled in the dark while struggling to remain mobile and keep a clear, sharp mindset focused on getting out of bed each morning, negotiating schedules, and showing up on time for lab work, diagnostic follow-up, and physician consultations. I learned to wear a brave face and present myself with dignity to demonstrate my life continued to be of value, not only to me, but also to my community.

On January 18th the drugs I needed were shipped finally to the CVS retail pharmacy where the whole process began. I retrieved my prescription and began taking the antivirals the following day. During the preceding week of confrontation, I figured out I should contact CVS Specialty Pharmacy no later than 7:35 a.m. (five minutes after customer service opened). Calls placed at that time seemed to be serviced within 15 minutes versus 60 to 90 minutes for later calls.

Wednesday, January 27 was my first appointment with Dr. Agha since my discharge from the hospital on Christmas Eve. Sitting in the small waiting room of his satellite clinic located within the Methodist Dallas Medical Center campus, my left brain function stepped through each permutation of treatment versus outcome. Absorbed in my own thoughts, some 15 minutes or so passed before I noticed the other people in the waiting room. To my right a few seats over, a young woman busied herself flipping through a magazine. Against the wall to my left sat an elderly man, leaning back with his eyes closed, breathing deliberately, and only occasionally waving his fingers slowly, his hands resting on a walking cane. Finally, I noticed a tired-looking middle-aged couple seated opposite me. I could see years of physical labor etched in their faces. The man stared into some invisible abyss, listless and unresponsive to the frenetic attention of the woman next to him. She spoke quietly to her mate as she fidgeted with the sleeve of his jean jacket. This odd couple cracked through the invisible wall I had erected around myself. Although I tried to avoid eavesdropping, it was impossible not to overhear what was said. "How long do you think we're going to have to wait?" the woman asked, looking at the time on her mobile phone, and gently shaking the man's arm. "We've been here 20 minutes already," she exclaimed, "and every 20 minutes costs us another dollar!" The young woman seated to my right was also eavesdropping, but unlike me, she had no qualms about it. She rose from her chair, crossed the room and stood in front of the whispering couple. She held out a yellow card, which she tried to give to the whispering woman. Returning to her seat, she continued her conversation with the couple aloud, for everyone to hear. "If you go down stairs to the first floor you'll see an information booth where you can get an application for one of these yellow cards. Fill that out and you will be issued a card that will validate your parking at any of the garages and you'll never have to pay more than one dollar." The young lady smiled, gesturing once again to the card. "It is good for a year, and you only need to fill out another form to renew it." Suddenly the listless man became animated as he struggled to stand. His steps were labored, but he walked as quickly as he could, as he left the waiting room, and disappeared down the hall.

Instinctively, I reached for my wallet, intent on withdrawing a $5 or $10 bill and offering it to the woman who fixed her gaze anxiously on the waiting room door – but I thought better of it. My noble intentions could be easily misinterpreted, ending in embarrassment for her *and* me. It would be best to wait and see how things played out on the first floor. But I couldn't help asking myself if the couple was really worried about the extra dollars they may have to pay for parking.

After several minutes the man returned, collapsing in the chair next to the woman. Again she grabbed the sleeve of his jacket, anxious to learn if he was successful in obtaining the parking validation card. He sighed heavily to catch his breath, and without saying a word, opened his hand to reveal a yellow card. The woman clutched the card to her chest as if it were a strand of pearls or a diamond bracelet. "I was so worried about how much we'd have to pay for parking. The longer we sit here the more it costs." She closed her eyes, nearly in tears as she breathed a heavy sigh of relief.

Wow! I had been totally absorbed in my own mental drama, wondering how I could elevate Dr. Agha's tenuous impression of me, while this unfortunate couple struggled with the prospect of paying a $5 parking fee. Would $5 mean less money for groceries or their pharmaceutical co-pay? How devastating would the accumulation of parking fees be should they need to return to this office several times within the month? Could a few dollars really be that important? Then I began to feel a bit guilty about my own financial circumstances. Even my disability income (60% of my standard take-home pay) was probably many times their regular income. A medical condition could devastate their lives. Although I faced a journey fraught with unknowns, in that moment I could see how truly blessed were my circumstances.

At that first meeting following my hospitalization, Dr. Agha's demeanor remained stiff and distant. I felt certain he was still under the impression that I was a lying drug user.

During our second meeting, he confirmed Dr. Brenner's analysis and told me my case had two separate profiles. The person described in the lab notes should be hospitalized, but the person seated in front of him retained a vibrant appearance. It would be necessary to treat both profiles simultaneously. Dr. Agha explained that the kidneys perform a variety of tasks in addition to filtering the blood. Another vital function is to secrete chemicals that catalyze the body's production of bone marrow, which in turn affects the production of red blood cells. When the kidneys are damaged they cannot secrete a sufficient amount of chemicals to stimulate the continued growth of those red blood cells, which carry oxygen throughout the body. The shortness of breath I experienced in May 2015 in Maui was likely a symptom caused by my severely damaged kidneys. Being able to rest during that vacation allowed my system to recover somewhat – the likely reason the shortness of breath abated.

When I visited Dr. Brenner on February 8th, she ordered blood work to check my viral loads as three weeks had passed since I began taking the antiviral cocktail. On my March visit I found her elated that the tests of the prior month confirmed my HIV viral load was undetectable. My hepatitis-B viral load had fallen to just over 7000. Dr. Brenner informed me that she had expected this particular therapy to require six months to a year before my viral loads would become undetectable. These results were unprecedented within a three-week time period – simply unheard of. She concluded my immune system and my overall excellent health had not only controlled the viruses for the previous 15 years, but also contributed to my body's miraculous response to the therapy.

Dr. Brenner's explanation for the misdiagnosis of my viral infections coupled with the effective therapy she prescribed offered a glimmer of hope, but it would take another month of close observation and blood analysis to convince Dr. Agha there was a course of treatment that could make me a viable candidate for a kidney transplant.

Working together, Drs. Agha, Brenner, and Chowdhury eventually were able to stabilize my system. In late March they reached consensus about the best way to proceed in preparation for kidney transplant. All affirmed my condition was survivable. Even so, it was not yet clear how resilient my physiology would be in response to the antiviral therapy or any future pharmacological strategies that may be required. Although there were still many unanswered questions, at least I had some assurance about the source of my kidney failure. I was by no means out of the woods, but a ray of sunlight finally made its way through the treetops.

Dr. Chowdhury agreed to be responsible for blood work and supervising the lab analyses requested regularly by Dr. Agha. I was pleased that this arrangement kept her in the loop, but her interest in my mental and psychological wellbeing was equally important. During our weekly conversations (by phone or in person), she fervently encouraged me to inform the people in my *circle of care* about my health challenges. She believed I needed their support to endure what was to come. My Myers-Briggs INTJ[3] personality profile confirmed me to be a very private and

---

[3] INTJ (introversion, intuition, thinking, judgment) is an abbreviation for one of sixteen psychological types defined in the Myers-Briggs Type indicator (MBTI) profiles. INTJs (aka: "The Architect") is a rare profile; forming just 2% of the population, and women of this personality type are especially rare, forming just 0.8% of the population – it is often a challenge for them to find like-minded individuals who are able to keep up with their relentless intellectualism and chess-like maneuvering. People with the INTJ personality type are imaginative yet decisive, ambitious yet private, amazingly curious, but they do not

introverted person. It was extremely difficult for me to step beyond my comfort zone and share my personal tragedy with others. I was uncomfortable with this level of transparency.

Then I imagined myself in JJ's position as he so boldly prompted me to bench myself from the employment game. I recalled from the beginning of our friendship he told me I needed to prioritize myself more often, rather than always placing myself last in line. As it turned out, a key decision affecting my treatment was accepting JJ's recommendation to go on short-term disability. I discovered that my mental and physical exhaustion had been masked by my insane work schedule, which started at 4 a.m. and ended at 6 p.m., Monday through Friday. My doctors told me eventually that it was critically important to remove myself from the constant low-level stress of my work environment. Doing so would accelerate my body's response to the therapies over the next several months. In that moment of reflection I experienced the first of many epiphanies. I realized JJ was my champion. It was my connection with him that prompted me to adopt my *healthy self-interest* philosophy. Even though our professional paths diverged ten years ago, he was still fighting for me. If this were possible, then how many other relationships had I misinterpreted?

This realization and my faith in Dr. Chowdhury led me to set aside my pride and reveal the dire condition of my health to my friends. Eventually, I realized sharing my medical crisis was an opportunity to experience deeper connections with them. *Ah hah!* There would be no downside to exploring these uncharted waters.

---

squander their energy. INTJs are able to live by glaring contradictions that nonetheless make perfect sense – at least from a purely rational perspective. For example, INTJs are simultaneously the most starry-eyed idealists and the bitterest of cynics, a seemingly impossible conflict. But this is because INTJ types tend to believe that with effort, intelligence and consideration, nothing is impossible, while at the same time they believe that people are too lazy, short-sighted or self-serving to actually achieve those fantastic results.

Reflecting on my face-off with the Dallas Fire Department in my tidy whities, I was finally able to laugh at the absurdity of my staunch intellection. At this point, only JJ knew I had been hospitalized during Christmas week. I made a short list of people to call, including my closest friends and associates – the people with whom I interacted most often.

I took a deep breath and began to make the calls. As I did so, I discovered people were quite angry with me for not trusting them with the knowledge that I had been hospitalized during the week of Christmas. My initial response was that I did not know enough about what was wrong to share any cogent information. I pointed out that my medical support team was struggling to understand what may be possible and prudent as a course of treatment, and that the combination of these unknowns left me unable to provide answers to any questions prior to March. A few accepted this as a logical explanation, but most thought I was full of bullshit. The latter was closer to the truth. In fact, I was embarrassed about not knowing how this happened to me. I did not know what I was going to do about it. And I was terrified that I would lose the people closest to me.

As I began living through the unfamiliar feelings of withdrawal from the stress of my aggressive work schedule, I had time for quiet reflection, which helped immensely. I began to navigate a significant learning curve as I acceded that my relationships with those in my *circle of care* were not solely under my control.

In all my 60 years I never allowed myself to believe it was possible for anyone other than my parents to give a tinker's damn about my life, nor was I aware that I added anything to anyone else's. Another epiphany came as I considered that my nuclear family survived in a virtual cocoon, which limited exposure to unwarranted attacks from the political and social strictures in Waterloo. My sister's social intelligence was stymied, I believe, as her allergies made it impossible for her to play outside like other children. For a different reason, mine also had been delayed. The cocoon in which our family existed left me capable only of cautious and distant friendships, and unable to believe my friends could truly care about me. At the same time, they were free to form their own personal connection with me, and the value they placed on that connection was largely beyond my knowledge or influence. I had not been free enough psychologically to trust in the resilience of these connections.

The anger expressed by my friends was not about my ignorance, but rather, that my actions had ignored the depth of their authentic care and concern for my well-being. Feeling encouraged, I made a second, longer list of friends with whom I interact less frequently. I drafted an email summarizing my diagnosis and prognosis, and broadcast that email to those on this list.

Dr. Chowdhury's counsel was indispensable. She was my champion from the very beginning. Dr. Brenner, my infectious disease specialist, was driven by test results. She demonstrated almost immediately a keen interest in my medical profile and physiological response to antiviral therapy. She expressed on several occasions her delight and astonishment with my consistently robust response to my medical care. Drs. Chowdhury and Brenner were caring. They saw me as a credible human being. They were clearly on my side.

I found Dr. Agha, my nephrologist, to be a challenge. His stoic and stern demeanor, coupled with his tenacious quest for precision and intellectual certainty, was not easily informed by intangibles. I knew from our initial meeting on Christmas Eve there was little trust between us. I thought he was a lunatic – that he had confused my lab results with some other wretched soul. In turn, I am certain he believed me to be a liar, chronic drug user, and promiscuous sexual deviant. Still, my life was in his hands. How could I to convince this premier medical expert that my character and life's work were significant and noble? What could I do to help him see me as a human being with a life worth saving? What could I do to encourage him to put his considerable expertise and influence to work on my behalf? I decided to allow science to build my case and contradict his negative assumptions about me.

I believed Dr. Brenner's explanation for my extremely low viral loads. The clinical evidence I did not have a live syphilis infection, would also help my case, but I needed more.

One morning in February I woke at 5 a.m. with a stark realization: Dr. Agha's first impression of me was as a depressed patient in a rumpled hospital gown, unshaven, unbathed, and hair uncombed. He knew nothing of my education, profession, or philanthropy. I would send him my curriculum vitae. I would also dress in a conservatively tailored gray suit and tie for my upcoming examination.

On the day of my next visit with Dr. Agha, my phone rang at 7:05 a.m. It was my buddy Jason from Kansas City, Kansas calling from his farm north of the city as dawn was breaking. "Reggie, I've been thinking about your email and woke up this morning with a strong urge to talk to you. I wanted to tell you that I've decided to donate my kidney for your surgery." My world stopped for moment. I was silent. Words failed me as I absorbed Jason's extraordinary offer. Before I asked how he came to this decision, Jason spoke again, "This is something I can do…something I want to do for you."

Later that same morning I received a phone call from my friend Mark in Plano, Texas. "Man, how are you doing? I got your email and I wanted you to know that I consider you to be family. Tell me what I need to do to donate my kidney for your surgery?"

What was going on? I wondered. I felt as though my world had been turned upside down and pulled inside out. I had not even *contemplated* asking anyone to become a donor.

I arrived at Dr. Agha's clinic that afternoon, following an evaluation by a vascular surgeon for catheterization in preparation for peritoneal dialysis. My creatinine levels were nearing the tip-over point indicating dialysis would be a prudent precaution. Peritoneal dialysis would be less stressful on my body and would facilitate travel and returning to work. Dr. Agha referred me to a surgical center across from the Dallas Methodist Health Center for the catheter insertion. That morning I had undergone sonograms and met with the surgeon who mapped out the particular procedure he would be using to prepare me for dialysis.

Dr. Agha was delayed for about 30 minutes. As this was unusual, I became concerned that something may be drastically wrong with my lab results. But when he entered the examination room he was unusually buoyant and upbeat. "My apologies. I was distracted by problems with our Internet service while attempting to transmit records for another of my patients. I'm sorry to have kept you waiting." He went directly to his computer screen and pulled up my lab results, and pivoted on his stool to face me. "Have you met with the surgeon to plan your catheterization?"

"Yes, I am just coming from his office. He completed his preliminary examination, and the surgical center will be contacting me in a few days to schedule the procedure."

"That's excellent, but I am going to call the surgeon and cancel the procedure." Still recovering from my angst surrounding his tardiness, I was completely taken off guard as I tried to *comprehend* what I thought was hearing. He continued, "Your creatinine levels have fallen significantly, and your other labs indicate your system is stabilizing. I believe it would be in your best interest to avoid dialysis. I'm going to try to get you transplanted preemptively, avoiding the negative impacts dialysis – even peritoneal dialysis – would have on your system. I will call the surgeon today and cancel the procedure."

"Well I have good news, too. I received two unsolicited offers of kidneys this morning, just hours before my appointment with the surgeon. I don't know how this impacts the anticipated transplant surgery, but I'm thinking having access to live donors may be a good thing."

"That's fantastic news! Yes, live donation would be the very best outcome, particularly with your healthy profile. I'm glad you are doing so well. Let's meet again in one month."

Dr. Agha enthusiastically encouraged me to register with the Dallas Methodist Hospital Kidney/Pancreas Transplant Center. He would have his assistant send me the application within the week. Once the application was submitted, I would be scheduled for a thorough prescreening later that spring.

Yes! Success! Compared to the adversarial tenor of our first meeting on Christmas Eve, and his reserved posture during our second meeting, I found Dr. Agha's change in attitude nothing short of amazing. He was genuinely excited about my prospects for kidney transplantation. I believe he now understood that I was as committed to my recovery as he and my other doctors. We definitely turned a significant corner in our relationship.

I left his office and walked across the parking lot to my car. But instead of immediately driving home, I just sat there for a few minutes in silence. I had struggled to break through the glass wall between Dr. Agha and me. I had been uncertain about sharing my situation with my friends, and beset by the uncertainty of my circumstances. I was still adjusting to withdrawal – not getting up at 4:30 and making the half-hour drive to work, and the one to two hour commute home. But today, not only had the glass wall around Dr. Agha been shattered, but also two of my friends offered their kidneys, and I would be considered formally for transplant surgery. This was too much good news to bear in one single day.

Each of my friends surrounded me with love and good wishes. Although not everyone offered me their kidney – LOL – each laid treasures of compassion, hope, support and goodwill at my feet. These offerings had no expiration date. March 18th I received a letter of acceptance for pre-evaluation from the Methodist Transplant Center, outlining an intense schedule of procedures, blood work, and doctors' consultations. The evaluation was scheduled to begin on April 12th and would continue for about 6 weeks. Within that 6-week window more good news found me. Carl, my trainer and close associate, became the third person to volunteer to be a kidney donor. This time I was not as stunned as I had been by the previous offers. I realized and accepted that these unsolicited offers were a testament to the depth of the connections I enjoyed among my "circle of care." I thought, *Perhaps I'll make it to the other side of this health crisis, after all.*

My parents always encouraged me to purchase quality goods and services. I frequented the same barber for over 30 years, retained Dr. Washington as my PCP for over 20 years, and the $400 black Bally loafers my mother gave me in 1975 are as supple and beautiful today as they were when I first wore them.

As well, since 1984 I have faithfully patronized the Uptown location of Faulkner's Fine Dry Cleaning. Established in 1954, Faulkner's is Dallas-based and family owned. The Uptown location employs many of the same people today as when I became a customer. My mother also purchased my first tuxedo at Neiman Marcus in 1975, which occasioned my first visit to Faulkner's. I left my tuxedo there to be cleaned, as they had come highly recommended. A couple of weeks later I returned to pick up the tux. The attendant took my claim check and quickly located my garment, which he handed over to me with an envelope, saying, "Mr. Harvey, we found this $184 cash inside the breast pocket of your jacket. We always check pockets before we process a garment, and we wanted to make certain we returned the money to you. We hope you are pleased with our service and look forward to seeing you again." That was the beginning of a beautiful friendship.

As my medical journey moved into summer, I suffered mobility setbacks due to a combination of gout and mild rheumatoid arthritis flare-ups. My kidney disease prevented taking acetaminophen or ibuprofen to control pain and swelling. My doctors were hesitant to prescribe anything that may interfere with my antiviral therapies and other drugs. In lieu of pain medication I learned to manage a strict diet, purchased a cane and learned to tolerate the pain in my feet, knees and hands. During this time I relied on friends to transport me to appointments and accompany me on errands. Occasionally I was able to drive my own car, which did wonders for my sense of mobility and independence.

Early one afternoon on the day I was scheduled to meet with Dr. Agha for a progress evaluation, I decided to retrieve my clothing from Faulkner's (dropped off previously by a friend) before heading to my appointment. The weather was particularly beautiful that day and I was determined to complete this errand on my own. As I parked at the drycleaners my attention was directed solely at opening my car door, getting my legs out from under the steering wheel onto the pavement, and determining how best to position for my cane to stand up and exit the car without falling. I had not been to Faulkner's for a while. The staff was concerned to see me struggling with that cane, and shocked I had lost so much weight. As I struggled with my uncertain choreography one of the attendants ran out of the store and came to my aid. "Mr. Harvey... It's so good to see you... Please just give me your claim check and credit card. I'll process your order and have someone place your clothes in the car. Just relax... I'll be right back." Before I had a chance to respond, the attendant had dashed back into the facility. Bewildered, I picked up my legs and swung them back underneath the steering wheel. I retrieved my cane, returned it in the passenger seat and lowered my window. I sat there – stunned at what had just transpired. I had not anticipated (nor did I want) any special treatment. How did the attendant even know it was me? I guess she recognized the car. Then I realized I had observed the staff address customers always by name as if each was a member of their family. So I guess it should have come as no surprise that they recognized my car. The attendant reappeared in short order with my receipt and credit card. Simultaneously another staffer opened the rear door and carefully placed my shirts and pants on the seat. Both attendants smiled, waved goodbye, and wished me a speedy recovery. I exited the parking lot and headed for my appointment with Dr. Agha.

I shared all this with the doctor and expressed my surprise at the kindness shown. Dr. Agha simply smiled, saying, "In this age of social media and self-absorption, it's nice to know that basic human kindness is still alive and well." I realized my preoccupation with my illness and my dogged determination to hang on to my independence rendered me oblivious, at times, to other offers of kindness, many from total strangers. I had no clue in my 30 years as a Faulkner's patron that I had become their friend.

On the last Friday in June my boss, JJ, called to inform me he was getting pressured from Human Resources to provide a formal, written job description for my position in the Infrastructure Architecture (IA) team. Evidently, UNUM (the CVS third-party benefit claims administrator) needed the job description to determine the physical and mental occupational demands of my job to assess the severity of my disability. Unable to find a copy of my job description in his archives, JJ asked if I had a copy that I could forward to him. I laughed, and reminded him that in October 2015 he and I collaborated to revise job descriptions for the entire IA team, but we never wrote descriptions for his position or mine. We both laughed. I suggested he dash off a summary of my responsibilities, but to my surprise he told me he preferred that I draft the job description and frame my responsibilities using the template we had designed for the rest of the team. He needed the document by Tuesday of the following week. I begrudgingly agreed to accept the task, and resolved to sacrifice my weekend to write the job description.

Bright and early Saturday morning I grabbed my company-issued laptop and initiated the standard login procedure, only to discover I had been locked out of the system. This seemed odd since I logged in the previous day to submit my weekly time sheet. I called Tech Support and learned that because of my extended absence, my security access had "expired", although my security profile was still current. Tech Support confirmed my security access could be reestablished, but to do so I needed to connect my laptop to a "live" docking station in the physical office. Because I had not used my electronic badge consistently since my leave, my 24 our building access was also rendered inactive. Therefore, I would need to wait until Monday when one of my IA teammates could provide me with access into building. I texted the IA team administrator and arranged a rendezvous for the following Monday at 6 a.m.

I arrived at my old office to find it had not yet been reassigned so I plugged my laptop into the docking station and called Tech Support. By 7 a.m. my security access to the Intranet was restored. I decided to complete the job description while in my office, as most workers would not begin rolling in until after 9 a.m. My plan was to complete the task and slip out before anyone noticed I was there. I did not relish answering an avalanche of questions. Summarizing the key roles of my position was simple, but enumerating the associated skills and responsibilities for each proved more challenging. The task took longer than I anticipated.

For the next four hours I assembled and reviewed the documentation before submitting it to JJ, per his instructions. Not until I packed up to leave the office did I realize how much time had passed. It was 11 a.m. Word had spread I was in the office. Over the next hour several of my IA colleagues came in to express how happy they were to see me. Each rolled the side chair as close to me as possible. Some leaned forward in the chair as if planning to place me in a bear hug. Others grasped my forearm in their hands. My personal space was assailed as they stared deeply in my eyes apparently in search of hidden clues. I heard, *Is this really*

Reggie?...He's lost so much weight!...Is he back to work for good?...Oh, my God, he's alive! My right-brain struggled to grasp the cascade of non-verbal cues, while my left-brain listened intently to the barrage of questions and the extensive briefings my colleagues volunteered. They seemed intent to fill in the 4-month gap since my leave of absence with an avalanche of data, which was of little use to me. I smiled involuntarily, declining their offers of assistance during my recovery.

Some shared the profound ways in which I had impacted their professional lives since I joined the team in 2011. I learned I had become the "go to" guy with whom they debated strategies, explored optimal solutions, defined task sequencing, and depended on for resourcing technical standards and new-hire orientation. I was the "Rosetta stone" for the team – the one to whom each came for advice, guidance, and reassurance. These were very smart and technically savvy people, each a seasoned expert in his or her domain. Having just completed a written autopsy of my team role, I saw clearly how they viewed my influence and impact as Advisor-Team Lead for Infrastructure Architecture (IA). I was humbled by the heart-felt concern and generosity expressed by colleagues whom I had not considered to be my friends.

Like many Americans, I was once under the illusion that health care insurance assures access to care and protects against the risk of incurring onerous medical expenses. Trying to use my insurance beyond annual physicals, inoculations, and such, has disabused me of this idea. Like a false prophet, indemnification (paid for on a monthly basis) may default on the promise of benefits, leaving one exposed to extensive financial risks, and even financial ruin.

As an employee of a Fortune 10 enterprise I was a privileged colleague among 250,000 workers. Certainly a group of this size enjoyed significant bargaining power regarding the terms of our group policy. I was rarely sick with anything more than a common cold or an occasional bout with the flu. I abhor paperwork and would never attempt to benefit from bogus insurance reimbursement schemes. I actively pursued preventative measures, adjusting to a healthier diet as I aged, maintaining a physical fitness routine, and getting a good eight hours' sleep. Each year I scheduled a physical examination. Even the discovery of my renal failure – alarming as it was – could not be blamed on a risky lifestyle.

My diagnosis was confirmed and documented by both my nephrologist and infectious disease specialist. So I believed that I had responsibly registered my catastrophic health condition adequately in my insurance claim profile. However, within the first 30 days of my medical leave I discovered my group insurance policy was separate from my group disability policy. I was not particularly concerned with this nuance – at least not in the beginning. Logic dictated that my renal failure was not self-repairable and that extraordinary measures (i.e., kidney transplant – and possibly dialysis) would be required to stabilize my health and prevent my death. These were medical facts – not suppositions. My naiveté about my insurance benefit would soon be shattered by reality.

My employer outsourced the administration of short-term disability claims to a third-party. I was assigned a primary caseworker, Matt, who introduced his role as my disability advocate. According to my group disability policy, I should expect a weekly stipend amounting to 60% of my gross income. With confirmation of my address, the weekly disability checks began to arrive in the mail. Every six weeks Matt called to check on "my well-being", and fax inquiries to my PCP, nephrologist and infectious disease specialist, requesting confirmation of my continued disability. The first two "wellness" checks were uneventful. But in the 18th week (just after my liver biopsy), the disability checks stopped coming. Matt called with his usual upbeat tone to inform me that upon review by their nurse, I was no longer eligible to receive disability benefits. Matt reported that my doctors' medical updates indicated that my system had stabilized. I reminded Matt that the primary reason I had been advised to take a medical leave was to remove myself from the stressful demands of my work. My resting blood pressure was closely monitored and was a critical factor for transplant approval. Matt's tone quickly became sarcastic. He explained, "Just because you are on a transplant list does not constitute confirmation of your physical disability."

I sat speechless and motionless. *What had this moron just said to me? Did he really just let those words across his lip? Really? Did he just say that?"* I could not engage in this illogical dialogue. After an uncomfortable silence Matt interjected, "Should you wish to challenge this decision, your doctors will need to send us an update of your medical condition." I simply hung up the phone, and sat quietly in my recliner. I thought back over the previous eight weeks, and recalled the transplant prequalification evaluation for which AETNA, my group health insurance provider, had just reimbursed the Dallas Methodist Health Center. During that evaluation I underwent: an electrocardiogram (EKG)[4]; a chest X-Ray (PA/LAT)[5]: an abdominal sonogram[6]; a Carotid Doppler[7]; an echocardiogram[8]; and a Myocardial Perfusion Scan (MPI)[9]. All this to determine if I could withstand the rigors of the transplant

---

[4] **EKG definition:** a test that checks for problems with the electrical activity of your heart.

[5] **PA/LAT definition:** the standard chest examination consists of a PA (posterior-anterior) and lateral chest x-ray; used to diagnose many conditions involving the chest wall, including its bones, and also structures contained within the thoracic cavity including the lungs, heart, and great vessels

[6] **Abdominal Sonogram definition:** a type of imaging test. It is used to look at organs in the abdomen, including the liver, gallbladder, spleen, pancreas, and kidneys. The blood vessels that lead to some of these organs, such as the inferior vena cava and aorta, can also be examined with ultrasound.

[7] **Carotid Doppler definition:** an imaging test that uses ultrasound to examine the carotid arteries located in the neck. This test can show narrowing or possible blockages due to plaque buildup in the arteries due to coronary artery disease.

[8] **Echocardiogram definition:** a test of the action of the heart using ultrasound waves to produce a visual display, used for the diagnosis or monitoring of heart disease.

[9] **Myocardial Perfusion Scan definition:** a nuclear medicine procedure that illustrates the function of the heart muscle (myocardium). It evaluates many heart conditions, such as

surgery preparation, operation and recovery. In addition, the pre-evaluation required numerous blood panels[10], and consults with the Dallas Methodist Health Center Liver Institute, the Director of Infectious Disease, and the Pancreas/Kidney Transplant Center cardiologist and transplant surgeon. Not only did the 8-week pre-evaluation confirm my need for a kidney transplant as soon as prudently possible, but it also established beyond question that I could not return to work before the transplant surgery and post-surgical recovery period concluded. Now this fool was telling me I needed to have my doctor send him an "update" to confirm my continued disability?

I called my PCP to schedule a visit to review Matt's request, and to formulate a strategy in collaboration with my nephrologist to provide irrefutable evidence of my medical condition. I left that consultation frustrated, angry and discombobulated, having lost confidence that my managed care benefits would see me through the transplant surgery.

A few days later I received another call from Matt. This time his voice was all ice cream and puppy dogs. His disposition was so sweet that I swear I developed cavities just listening to his babble. "Mr. Harvey, I'm calling to report we have received new information that allowed us to review your case once again. Were you aware that you also hold a private disability insurance policy?" *Of course I am aware of that, you imbecile*, I thought to myself. Several weeks before Matt informed me I was ineligible for continued short-term disability benefits, I received an odd call from a different office within the third-party disability administrative agency. A very nice and professional lady explained that she was the assigned long-term disability administrator. She explained my policy would begin to pay benefits 180 days following my original date of declared disability (February 12, 2016). In

---

coronary artery disease (CAD), hypertrophic cardiomyopathy and heart wall motion abnormalities.

[10] NOTE: during one such blood draw the phlebotomist withdrew 17 vials of blood.

mid-August the policy benefit would activate and I should expect to receive an additional $1000 each month thereafter. Matt droned on, "The office that administers your private disability insurance policy functions completely separate from our role as administration for your short-term group disability coverage. That office conducted a separate review of your medical history and physician notes, and has filed an opinion that enabled us to review your case." I chuckled to myself, thinking *"Aha, you've been caught with your pants around your ankles – and to cover your ass, you're trying to convince me that out of the goodness of your heart you were able to offer a different interpretation of the medical history you so readily dismissed last week."* I provided Matt no indication of my attitude about his epiphany. Matt continued, "I am so happy to report that we will be issuing a check for the six weeks of disability benefit that had previously been withheld, and we will be paying the weekly benefit as originally scheduled through August 12, 2016 – or until you are cleared to return to work – whichever occurs first. Mr. Harvey, I hope that your health continues to improve."

I immediately called my PCP to relay the news that my disability benefit had been restored. I apologized for the inconvenience and abuse of time this unexpected disruption had caused Drs. Chowdhury and Agha. Dr. Chowdhury very kindly assured me no apology was expected or required. "Reggie, this is a game in which you don't get to learn the rules until you begin to play."

For the next four months my attention was consumed as I worked with Dr. Agha, to determine a prudent course of action to address my developing anemia. He explained that due to the extremely low function of my kidneys, my body believed it was being attacked by foreign bacteria and had ceased to process iron from my food intake. Iron resistance evolved as a defense mechanism stemming from the devastating plagues of the first millennium CE. None of the iron in the food I ate would be absorbed by my system – no matter how much I consumed. Evidently, bacteria depend on iron as a primary food source. Depriving bacteria of iron will starve the bacteria. A certain percentage of the population developed this defense mechanism and survived the plagues. Those who did not develop this mechanism died. It was crucial that another method be employed to restore my iron intake and retention sufficiently to nourish my bone marrow so that my body could produce the necessary red blood cells to efficiently sustain oxygen levels within my circulatory system. Otherwise, my stamina would continue to diminish and other serious health issues would interfere with my ability to withstand the transplant surgery. Dr. Agha consulted with a hematologist at the Texas Oncology Center, and the two agreed to perform intravenous infusions of iron sucrose weekly for a period of six weeks. Following these infusions my blood would be tested to see if my system was capable of sustaining appropriate levels of iron.

On Friday August 12, 2016 I received my fifth iron infusion. The following Monday I received a call from the Dallas Methodist Medical Center inquiring if there had been a change in my insurance. I reported that I was unaware of any change, and that my group health insurance policy had been renewed as of June 1st. But I agreed to check with my employer as an exercise in prudence. I called CVS Health human resources and was informed that because my short-term disability status was being converted to long-term disability, I was no longer considered an "active" employee; therefore my group insurance plan had been terminated on August 12th. I asked why I had not been given prior notification, and was told that I would be receiving written notification by mail within the next 7 to 10 days. "And how is that supposed to help me?" I asked. "I have not yet completed the iron infusion therapies to arrest my anemia, and the treatment will be suspended if I cannot provide proof of insurance." The representative seemed unmoved by the crisis posed by this "standard policy and procedure." The agent droned along, "Well, Mr. Harvey, you can apply for Consolidated Omnibus Budget Reconciliation Act (COBRA) coverage." Silence. "How do I do that? Where do I find instructions on the application process? How long will this take. What will this cost me?" I had seen nightmarish reports that COBRA premiums could run as high as $1500 per month per individual. I panicked! "Well, sir, I can apply for the COBRA on your behalf. In fact, I'm entering that information into the system as we speak. We have a special COBRA policy for long-term disability employees that will only increase your customary monthly premium by $50-$60 per month. Given that your "active" employee group health insurance plan terminated mid-month, you will have to pay the August and September total premium in one lump sum (approximately $1050) no later than October 1st or your health insurance will be permanently terminated. "OK, I'm prepared to pay that today. Can you help me process the transaction on this call?" "I'm sorry, Mr. Harvey. You can only pay that premium online at your employee HR online portal; and you can't pay it until it is actually billed to you on October 1."

I could feel my blood pressure beginning to boil over. "What do you mean I can't pay it now? What am I supposed to do in the meantime?" The HR representative remained pleasant, but detached and not forthcoming. "Sir, once you receive written notice that your 'active' employee group insurance plan has terminated, and once your October 1st premium is paid, the COBRA insurance will kick in retroactively as of August 13th. Any claims from health service vendors that are submitted after August 12th and before October 1st will simply have to be resubmitted for review and processing after the COBRA policy activates. "That's more than six weeks from now," I exclaimed. "I can't believe there is nowhere I could have read in advance about this 'standard policy and procedure' to terminate my insurance coverage in the middle of treatment for a near fatal medical condition. Begging your pardon, I'm not angry with you – I appreciate your being able to explain what's going on. However, for me this is a nightmare." "Mr. Harvey, that's just how it works. You should be receiving your policy termination letter in the mail within the next 7 to 10 days. Sometime after that, you will receive separate written notification concerning your transition to the COBRA policy. If it's any consolation to you, that COBRA policy will be exactly the same as the AETNA/Texas group insurance policy you had. The group number will be the same – as will the member number."

I hung up the phone, a technique I perfected in my previous inane conversations with Matt. I quickly typed up a summary of the so-called "standard policy and procedure" about which I had just been briefed, including the significant trigger dates and instructions regarding the process of resubmitting claims for payment. I spent eight hours of the next business day driving around the Dallas Metroplex to all of my health service providers to deliver my typed summary in person and discuss this unanticipated "transition" of my health insurance. Fortunately, the business office at the Texas Oncology Center where I was receiving the iron sucrose infusions was able to update their systems with the information I provided, and to my surprise I was able to avert interruption of the infusions.

This therapy proved very effective. To be certain, the hematologist recommended I also receive Darbepoetin Alfa shots every two weeks to balance out my hemoglobin (HGB) levels, which had fallen to an unhealthy level of 9. It was critical to raise my HGB level to 11 to prevent the need for blood transfusions. However, AETNA would have to pre-approve the shots. If preapproval were denied, another strategy would need to be employed. Fortunately, AETNA agreed to pay for the shots, which were billed at a rate of $5,000 per injection. My blood would be tested prior to the administration of the shot to monitor my HGB levels. When the levels stabilized above "11", the shots could be discontinued. Again, it was my good fortune that this insurance nightmare was contained, and my health service providers all agreed to ride the roller coaster with me. However, I maintained a kind of hypervigilance as I kept Dr. Chowdhury's words in mind: "This is a game in which you don't get to learn the rules until you begin to play."

I continued to improve over the summer and early fall. Several times during my appointments, Dr. Agha expressed his delight in the follow-up calls he was receiving from Dr. Chowdhury. He commented that she made an effort to reach out to his office every two weeks to provide updates on my overall care, and seek his advice about nuances of my treatment. Dr. Agha noted that Dr. Chowdhury's consistency made his job much easier and less stressful. With this I got the idea that perhaps it would be good if I could arrange for Dr. Chowdhury and Dr. Agha to meet face to face. I had an afternoon appointment scheduled with Dr. Agha on Wednesday, October 5th and decided to invite Dr. Chowdhury to accompany me if the scheduling worked out. About two weeks prior to my appointment, Dr. Chowdhury confirmed that indeed the date would work. I pondered whether to notify Dr. Agha of Dr. Chowdhury's intention to accompany me, but I decided against advance notice. I would allow the situation to unfold organically.

Dr. Chowdhury and I travelled together to Dr. Agha's office. Upon our arrival I introduced Dr. Chowdhury to Dr. Agha's nursing coordinator before we were led to the examination room. After about five minutes Dr. Agha burst into the room – grinning from ear to ear. "Oh, you must be Dr. Chowdhury. My nurse told me you were here! This is so fantastic!" He crossed the room with his hands outstretched to Dr. Chowdhury, and invited her to stand up from her chair. "Come with me – I want to introduce you to the other doctors in the clinic!" With that Dr. Agha excitedly escorted Dr. Chowdhury from the examination room. They disappeared for about 10 minutes. When they returned, Dr. Agha looked at me and said, "This never happens. It's unusual for a patient's PCP to make the time to accompany the patient to the examination with another doctor. But I'm so impressed that you made the time to accompany Reggie. He is my favorite patient, and I am personally biased about his outcome. I have recused myself from the transplant committee at Dallas Methodist because I am too invested in his care to be objective. It is the role of the transplant committee to give final approval for the live donor. And I just cannot in good conscience be a part of that decision because I want this transplant to happen tomorrow, if possible"

We all spoke for a few more minutes before Dr. Chowdhury and I left for the drive back to her office. Dr. Chowdhury was excited that Dr. Agha had introduced her with such zeal to his colleagues. He encouraged them all to join him in visiting Dr. Chowdhury's practice within the next few weeks. He suggested they collaborate closely with Dr. Chowdhury's practice, as it represented an exceptional and rare level of medical care.

I smiled broadly as Dr. Chowdhury recounted her visit with Dr. Agha and with his colleagues. I was pleasantly surprised to hear him declare that I – Reggie Harvey – had become his "favorite" patient. We had come very far indeed since our first meeting that fateful Christmas Eve almost a year ago.

My first two donors were not a match. However, Dr. Agha called on Friday, October 10 to inform me that my third "directed living donor"[11] and I were ABO[12] blood type mismatched, but our blood mismatch was "minimal." Dr. Agha indicated he spent the past week analyzing my transplant profile data, and had decided to

---

[11] **Directed living donor** definition: This term refers to a living individual willing to make a direct commitment to donate a kidney to a specific individual. Contrastingly, a "non-directed" living donor refers to people who volunteer to donate a kidney without naming any intended recipient.

[12] **ABO** definition (*Encyclopedia Britannica*): The ABO blood group system is the classification of human blood based on the inherited properties of red blood cells (erythrocytes) as determined by the presence or absence of the antigens A and B, which are carried on the surface of the red cells. Persons may thus have type A, type B, type O, or type AB blood. The A, B, and O blood groups were first identified by Austrian immunologists Karl Landstener in 1901.

Blood containing red cells with type A antigen on the surface has in its serum (fluid) antibodies against type B red cells. If, in transfusion, type B blood is injected into persons with type A blood, the red cells in the injected blood will be destroyed by the antibodies in the recipient's blood. In the same way, type A red cells will be destroyed by anti—A antibodies in type B blood. Type O blood can be injected into persons with type A, B, or O blood unless there is incompatibility with respect to some other blood group system also present. Persons with type AB blood can receive type A, B, or O blood.

propose the three best transplant options available to me.

The first option is called Kidney Paired Donation (KPD). About one third of people who offer to donate a kidney will be either blood type incompatible or human leukocyte antigen (HLA) incompatible with their intended recipient. Kidney paired donation (KPD), or kidney exchange, circumvents the incompatibility between donor and intended recipient by redistributing organs among two or more donors before the transplants. In the simplest type of KPD, two donors exchange kidneys so that their two candidates can each receive a compatible transplant. The donor operations are usually started simultaneously to prevent the situation in which one donor decides not to donate after that donor's intended recipient has already received a kidney.[13]

An expanded definition of KPD includes exchanges among three or more pairs. The donor of one pair gives the recipient of the next pair, whose donor gives to the recipient of the next pair, and so on, until the last pair's donor gives to the recipient of the first pair in the cycle. Moving to three-way or larger exchanges significantly increases the likelihood that any pair will find a match.

Many extensions to this concept, such as three-way and larger exchanges, compatible paired donation, and use of non-directed (altruistic) donors, have allowed greater numbers of people to find matches. KPD is the fastest-growing modality of living donation in the U.S., growing from just a handful of transplant in 2000 to surpass 500 transplants per year in 2010.[14] Kidney exchange accounted for nearly 10% of living kidney transplants in 2011.

The National Organ Transplantation Act of 1984 prohibits acquiring or transferring

---

[13] R.A. Montgomery et al., "Clinical Results From Transplanting Incompatible Live Kidney Donor/Recipient Pairs Using Kidney Paired Donation," *JAMA* 294, 13 (2005): 1655–1663.

[14] P. I. Terasaki, D. W. Gjertson, J. M. Cecka, "Paired Kidney Exchange Is Not A Solution To ABO Incompatibility," *Transplantation* 65, 2 (1998): 291.

a kidney for valuable consideration. Therefore, members of the transplant community pressed the U.S. Congress to pass the Charlie W Norwood Living Organ Donation Act of 2007 – clarifying that kidney exchange was legal. The current landscape for KPD in the U.S. includes several single-center programs,[15] multicenter consortia,[16] and the registry operated by the organization that administers deceased donation in the U.S., the United Network for Organ Sharing (UNOS).

Methodist Specialty and Transplant Hospital (San Antonio) has the largest KPD program in the U.S. By using sophisticated computer software, the team provided matches to 134 patients between 2008 and 2011. The San Antonio team has provided more kidney paired donation (KPD) transplants than any other single-center in the nation. The program has been especially effective in helping patients that statistically would not be a match with 80-100 percent of the population because of the antibodies in their blood; previous kidney transplants and pregnancy can result in a complicated string of antibodies that can result in organ rejection.

Dr. Agha is the former medical director of the San Antonio program. With the KPD option, my "directed" live donor would donate his kidney via the San Antonio facility and they in turn would match me with a perfectly compatible live kidney donor selected from the KPD registry.

The second option offered by Dr. Agha is called *desensitization*. In a new study

---

[15] A. W. Bingaman et al., "Single-Center Kidney Paired Donation: the Methodist San Antonio Experience," *American Journal of Transplantation* 12, 8 (2012): 2125–2132.

[16] Multiple references:
- F. L. Delmonico, "Exchanging Kidneys – Advances in Living-Donor Transplantation," *New England Journal of Medicine* 350, 18 (2004): 1812–1814.
- J. Veale, G. Hil, "National Kidney Registry: 213 Transplants in Three Years," *Clinical Transpl*antation (2010): 333–344.
- S. K. Akkina et al., "Donor Exchange Programs In Kidney Transplantation: Rationale And Operational Details From The North Central Donor Exchange Cooperative," *American Journal of Kidney Disease* 57,1 (2011): 152–158.

published Wednesday (03/09/2016) in *The New England Journal of Medicine*, Dr. Agha successfully altered patients' immune systems to allow them to accept kidneys from incompatible donors. Significantly more of those patients were still alive after eight years than patients who had remained on waiting lists or received a kidney transplanted from a deceased donor. Desensitization[17] "has the potential to save many lives," said Dr. Jeffrey Berns, a kidney specialist at the University of Pennsylvania's Perelman School of Medicine and president of the National Kidney Foundation.

Desensitization might be viewed as an alternative to KPD. However, some incompatible pairs can only be transplanted through a combination of desensitization and KPD. This situation arises when a transplant candidate has very high donor-specific antibody levels against the intended donor, but the candidate has a lower level of donor-specific antibody for some other donor in the exchange pool. Often patients are told their living donor is incompatible, so they are stuck on waiting lists for a deceased donor – sometimes for years; and a considerable number of patients waiting on cadaver donor lists die before being successfully matched.

Dr. Agha would adjust my blood chemistry to "match" my "designated" donor's ABO blood profile – thus suppressing any organ rejection due to ABO incompatibility. Desensitization involves first filtering the antibodies out of a patient's blood. The patient is then given an infusion of other antibodies to provide some protection while the immune system regenerates its own antibodies. "For some reason – exactly why is not known – the patient's regenerated antibodies are less likely to attack the new organ," says Dr. Dorry Segev (the lead author of the new study and a transplant surgeon at the Johns Hopkins University School of

---

[17] Desensitization: Protocols using high-dose intravenous immunoglobulin (IVIg) or plasmapheresis and low-dose IVIg have enabled successful transplants against either human leukocyte antigen (HLA) or blood type incompatibilities.

Medicine). But if the patient's regenerated natural antibodies are still a concern, the patient is treated with drugs that destroy any white blood cells that might make antibodies that would attack the new kidney.

The desensitization procedure takes time – for some patients as long as two weeks – and is performed before the transplant operation, so patients must have a living donor. The process is expensive, costing $30,000, and uses drugs not approved for this purpose. The transplant (by comparison) costs about $100,000. But kidney specialists agree that desensitization is cheaper in the long run than dialysis, which costs $70,000 a year for life.

Option three was to register with the Johns Hopkins "Hope Act" Transplant Study.[18] In February 2016 Johns Hopkins University received approval from the United Network for Organ Sharing (UNOS) to be the first hospital in the U.S. to perform HIV+ to HIV+ organ transplants. "This is an unbelievably exciting day for our hospital and our team, but more importantly for patients living with HIV and end-stage organ disease. For these individuals, this means a new chance at life," says Dr. Dorry Sergev, Associate Professor of surgery at Johns Hopkins University School of Medicine. In March 2016 Johns Hopkins performed two HIV-positive to HIV-positive kidney transplant surgeries; both with positive results. Johns Hopkins will remain the primary Hope Act clinical trial hospital, but several transplant centers have been approved to participate, in particular, the Pancreas/Kidney Transplant program at Dallas Methodist Medical Center.

Approximately 122,000 people are on the U.S. transplant waiting list at any one

---

[18] The HIV Organ Policy Equity (HOPE) Act (enacted on November 21, 2013) calls for the development and publication of research criteria relating to transplantation of HIV+ organs into HIV+ individuals. By November 21, 2015 the secretary of Health and Human Services (HHS) must revise the section of the organ procurement and transplantation network (OPTN) final rule (42 CFR 121.6) to enable the OPTN to adopt and use standards to recover of HIV + organs (from deceased donors) for kidney transplantation. This research is being done to learn whether organ transplantation from HIV-positive deceased donors is as safe and effective in HIV-positive recipients as transplants from HIV-negative deceased donors.

time. Thousands die each year, many of whom may have lived had they gotten the organ they needed. Meanwhile, Segev estimates that each year, about 500 to 600 HIV-positive would-be donors had organs that could have saved more than 1000 people – if only the medical community had been allowed to use the organs for transplant.

There is a higher risk of rejection of the new organ in HIV-positive patients, but nothing is known about rejection of organs from HIV-positive donors. This is one of the reasons the "Hope Act" study is being conducted. If one agrees to participate in this study, one can receive organ offers from HIV+ deceased donors for transplant. The participant will also remain on the standard organ waitlist.

One idea about this is that the medicines used to control HIV may interfere with the medicines used to avoid rejection of the new organ. In order to avoid this risk, HIV medicines that may cause this problem will be avoided whenever possible. Rejection medicines will be picked that are individual to the study participant that may lessen the chance of rejecting the new organ.

In African-American kidney transplant patients with HIV, some doctors have found the form of a gene (APOL1) related to kidney disease. "Now that the importance of the gene is known, clinicians could potentially genotype — or map the genes — of African Americans with chronic kidney disease (CKD) to assess their risk for disease progression," said Afshin Parsa, M.D., a nephrologist at the University of Maryland School of Medicine in Baltimore and a CRIC Study investigator. "This discovery provides direct evidence that African-Americans with established CKD and the APOL1 risk gene variant experience a faster decline in kidney function compared to their white counterparts, irrespective in most cases of what caused their kidney disease."

In late September 2016, I was invited to consider being one of five participants through the Pancreas/Kidney Transplant program at Dallas Methodist Medical

Center. Should I be unable to proceed with desensitization or the KPD program in San Antonio, Dr. Agha is reserving as an option his approval of my participation in the Hope Act clinical study.

Dr. Agha called me back around 2 p.m. on Friday, October 28th to inform me he had spoken with the medical director at the San Antonio Methodist Specialty and Transplant Hospital. He was assured the San Antonio KPD program would accept my case, despite the double viral infections (HIV and hepatitis B). Dr. Agha was confident that these were my best three options for transplant. He was convinced that I would successfully complete either the KPD matching and/or desensitization within the next few months. He asked and received my permission to forward my contact information to the admissions office in San Antonio.

Dr. Agha was willing to leverage his professional relationships to aggressively seek the best outcomes for my transplant surgery. We had formed a bond of trust and mutual respect. It was such a good feeling to enjoy affinity and comradery among my entire medical team: Dr. Chowdhury, Dr. Brenner and finally, Dr. Agha.

10 Hawaii with Cassandra

At this writing, Christmas 2016 is just five weeks away. I can hardly believe nearly a year has passed since I began my roller coaster ride through the nightmare of insurance providers, pharmaceutical services and managed care. Looking back at the preceding ten months I realize I showed up for no fewer than 34 doctor visits, had my blood drawn 22 times and experienced 9 medical procedures. Furthermore, I waged countless battles with my short-term disability insurance administrators, including the horror story of negotiating to re-instate my group health insurance, which was terminated without advance notice. By the end of May – about halfway through the aforementioned medical events – I was mentally and psychologically exhausted.

During February, while my survival was still an open question, I scheduled an escape to Maui without consulting anyone, including my doctors. I hoped and prayed I would be alive to make the journey set for my 61st birthday. I completed in mid-May the second and final phase of my transplant surgery pre-evaluation. Apart from my ongoing struggle with rheumatoid arthritis, my health was stable. During a May 11th examination, Dr. Agha determined my creatinine levels precluded the immediate need for dialysis, and my viral infections remained undetectable. When I met with Dr. Chowdhury two days later, I thought it prudent to seek her opinion about my planned respite from the pressures and responsibilities inherent in my role as a patient. Dr. Chowdhury thought my trip would be therapeutic, but she was a bit concerned about me travelling alone. I assured her that I had arranged to travel with my friend, Cassandra. A few weeks earlier I arranged a dinner to introduce Dr. Chowdhury to Cassandra and the rest of "The Crew", my posse of contemporaries who keep me grounded. I wanted her to meet the people she encouraged me to invite along on my medical saga. Dr. Chowdhury was confident I would be in capable hands. So at 7 a.m. Sunday, May 22, Cassandra and I boarded a first-class direct flight from Dallas to Maui, and my escape from reality began!

After takeoff we settled in for the eight-hour flight. Like children examining new toys, we played with the seats, which were equipped with the latest movie, sound, and lighting, and converted at the touch of a button to a sleeping berth. The most complicated apparatus was the food trays. After a couple of glasses of Cabernet and Merlot, we relaxed for the first time in months, allowing our hectic worlds be absorbed by the low hum of the twin GE CF6 Turbofan engines. Finally I could exhale, casting off the weight of constant vigilance and stress created by the need to respond at a moment's notice to a call from a physician, insurance agent, nursing coordinator or pharmacist. I was *free*!

I donned my new noise-canceling headphones and plugged into the extensive music collection on my Kindle device. As the music began to soothe my soul I casually rolled my head to the side and opened my eyes to watch Cassandra sipping her Cabernet and casually thumbing through a fashion magazine. I closed my eyes and thought about the person sitting next to me, whom I met in 2009 when we were seated next to each other at a charity luncheon. We began a conversation that continues to this day. In the ensuing years I observed her to be an astute businesswoman with a brilliant-cut diamond personality. She does not simply enter a room, but she swoops in like the *Scandal* heroine Elizabeth Pope, in full diva mode. Cassandra was simply gorgeous. Without trying, she drew the attention of men and women alike. Women, to measure their own fashion sense against her stunning image, and men, to perform the most difficult platform dives to win her attention. But all quickly found Cassandra to be delightfully and authentically, just Cassandra. She couldn't help it. That's just who she is. Listening to the lull of those Turbofan engines I caught my breath slightly as I realized this fabulous woman had set aside eight days on her unremitting calendar to act as my companion (and caregiver, if necessary).

Cassandra was the first person I told of my Christmas Eve hospitalization and diagnosis. She invited me to dinner in her home for the holidays. It was totally out of character for me to discuss something so personal, not to mention life-threatening, but I found myself divulging involuntarily my medical quandary over salmon and asparagus. I guess I just needed to tell someone. Following that holiday dinner, Cassandra called me every night to inquire about my well-being. As my medical team grappled with the best course of action, there was something special about her persistence and sincerity in those calls. No less than once a week she appeared graciously at my door to insist that I accompany her to afternoon cocktails or early evening dinners at some fabulous venue. Every valet, maître d' and sommelier seemed to know her, and welcomed her warmly. Just a flash from her intoxicating smile sent them on an endless quest to make us feel at home. Regardless of my pain or my waning energy level, Cassandra refused to allow me to find solace in some dark space. She would just toss my ass in that gorgeous black Mercedes and whisk me off to wondrous adventures and back home again. When necessary, she got out of her car, took hold of my arm and helped me climb those 17 steps to my front door. Often she carried my bags up those stairs, talking buoyantly the entire time, making me feel like a whole and well person despite my infirm state. I have no idea what spurred her to do this for me, but during the weeks and months following my disclosure, Cassandra helped me to look beyond my walls to the depth of the connections I enjoyed within my circle of care. It was truly humbling that she extended such ardent concern for my wellbeing.

We engaged in excited conversations about our anticipated adventures in paradise. Both of us had reached milestones in our work and personal lives, and this trip represented a homage to our frenzied pasts and more promising futures. This suspension of time would allow us to breathe deeply – to reset our mental and physical auras in support our dreams and aspirations.

Our flight landed at 2:30 p.m. Sunday. As we disembarked we were caressed by the fresh and fragrant air of the Pacific Ocean. We collected our luggage, boarded the resort shuttle and finally we were en route to our destination, a 26-acre resort on Maui's northwest shore. Although chatty during the previous hour, Cassandra fell silent as we made the one-hour drive to the resort. She seemed transfixed by the blue, green, and yellow hues of the midday ocean as the waves gently crashed upon the shore along the coastal highway. I heard only occasional sighs and utterances of awe: *"Oh, my God … look at that."* Eventually we reached our destination, crossing the threshold of the exquisite north lobby lanai. The ocean view was filled with fragrant and exotic fauna, while Koi swam along lazily in the Canals crisscrossing the campus.

I made my way to one of the check-in stations and watched as Cassandra worked her magic. She floated across the floor in her white short-shorts, white woven wedge heels and a colorful silk wrap. There it was: that brilliant-cut diamond smile. It is amazing that for all the attention Cassandra attracts, she manages to channel that positive energy and radiate it back to those she encounters. She can have a conversation with just a glance and a smile. Observing her fall into a natural rhythm, I thought, *the Westin Ka'anapoli will never be the same*. I turned my attention to the agent, focusing on the concierge itinerary and suite features requested and confirmed with my reservation. Cassandra diverted her path toward the sparkling freshwater stand. The reservation agent smiled broadly, looking at me (or so I thought), and said "Welcome, Mrs. Harvey. We, the concierge staff at the Ka'anapoli Ocean Villas welcome you and sincerely hope you will avail yourself of our services to improve your experience as our guest!"

Mrs. Harvey? Where ... What ... Who was he addressing? I quickly snapped my gaze behind me to find Cassandra standing there with two cups of ice-cold water garnished with lemon, lime, and mango. Here gaze slowly met mine. We both had this questioning look on our faces and then burst into quiet laughter. Apparently, the staff assumed she and I were a couple; that she was my wife. We would play along. Why not? I accepted the fruit-infused water she offered. "Thank you, dear," I said. *Lights! Camera! Action!* Our sitcom was officially in production. The agent presented me with the access cards, which I handed to our waiting valet who led us to our suite.

Our "home" for the next eight days was nestled in the corner on the top floor. The 1000 square foot space housed a galley kitchen framed by a breakfast bar, dining room, a living room with a queen-sized sofa bed, a separate king-sized bedroom, a luxurious spa bathroom and a laundry room. There was a spacious lanai off the living area. We quickly agreed we could *suffer* the week in this luxurious setting. We would visit markets the next day to supply our needs for snacks and light meals.

We rested a couple of hours before heading into the town of Lahaina for a 7 p.m. dinner reservation at Mala, a quaint family-owned bistro nestled on a rocky inlet continuously pounded by white frothy waves. Cassandra wore a figure-flattering sky blue dress accessorized with a turquoise and silver statement necklace. Naturally, the restaurant staff and several guests flocked toward her throwing compliments like flowers at her feet. We were seated promptly at a corner table. Through the open windows we could feel a soft ocean breeze and hear the pounding surf. I ordered a Merlot. Cassandra requested a Mai Tai. We downed our cocktails quickly and ordered a second round. This time Cassandra drank slowly, savoring the freshness of her drink. Suddenly, a bejeweled sunset burst through on the horizon, screaming with vivid blues, reds, and yellows, and cascading its shimmering light across the ocean surface toward our perch in the bistro. With this, Cassandra froze for moment and slowly turned toward me. "I'm not sure if it's this Mai Tai or my imagination, but I think I just saw God's arm fall from the sky and touch the water!" In Maui, God's Crayola® box holds 64 colors – not eight – many of which we cannot spell or pronounce. It must be a combination of the latitude and the tilt of the earth's axis in late spring that plays this trick on the eyes. A Maui sunset is incomparable. Cassandra took one more sip of her Mai Tai and raised her glass to toast the sky. "Yep, God lives here."

Monday morning we woke just as the sun was beginning to rise. As Cassandra opened the sliding glass doors to the lanai to let in a burst of that sweet, fragrant air, she announced plans to don her sneakers and go for an early morning walk along the beach. A five-mile path around the resort is dotted with macadamia trees and runs along the pristine white sand beach. We agreed to meet up around 7:30 on the south side of the resort for breakfast. I had slept deeply and I felt absolutely wonderful. After about an hour I got up, showered, and dressed in an extra-long gray T-shirt and green and gray board shorts. If I wanted to go swimming hour or so after breakfast, I did not want to walk all the way back to our suite to change clothes. It was a beautiful morning, about 76 degrees with a mild ocean breeze. Recovering from a flare-up a few days earlier of rheumatoid arthritis, I was happy to be able to walk now with minimal support from my cane. I put on my Crocs and struck out for the buffet breakfast. It was wonderful to be mobile again, and the warm sun felt so good against my skin. I was in no particular hurry as I tackled each gentle hill along the path, taking on the last one with ease and finding myself between two low-standing palm trees. My mouth watered as I anticipated the taste of fresh, sweet strawberries and pineapple for breakfast, but my musing was interrupted. *Oh ... my ... God*, I thought in horror, as my shorts slipped from my hips and fell to my ankles. Even my extra-long T-shirt did not shield me from the caress of the ocean breeze blowing between my legs and up my backside. In terror, I stopped in my tracks, threw down my cane and stooped over to retrieve the errant garment. I looked around to see if any wandering eyes – especially those belonging to children – caught sight of the mishap. Thankfully, no one had. Although these shorts fit snuggly last year, I now found it necessary to adopt the pose of teenagers who "sag" while sporting designer underwear. In that instant, *sagging* held less appeal for me than ever. Who wants to walk around with a fistful of trousers? Evidently I failed to appreciate the impact of shedding 50 pounds in five months. I stooped to retrieve my cane and carefully finished my jaunt to breakfast.

I found Cassandra seated comfortably at her table hiding behind huge sunglasses and munching on fresh fruit.

"Oh, babe ... you finally made it. I was just about to call you."

"I had a slight wardrobe malfunction at the top of that last hill over there," I said, gesturing behind me.

"What? A wardrobe malfunction?" I quickly told her of the incident, only to duck the strawberry she spit across the table in gut-busting laughter.

"That's not funny."

"Yes, the hell it *is* funny! I volunteered to help you this trip, but I'm drawing the line at the striptease act."

"Hush. With an attitude like that, this marriage will end in divorce before the week is up!"

We both fell back in our chairs and laughed again. After several glasses of that fabulous fresh water and raspberry iced tea, we gorged ourselves on more strawberries, pineapple, mango, and bacon. Stuffed, we agreed to stitch our fantasy marriage back together – for the sake of the resort staff.

Throughout the week we explored activities within the Ka'anapoli Ocean Villas, a town within a town, offering 14 residential buildings, pools, beaches, restaurants and markets. We rented a car and took several excursions around the island, making a point to spend a lazy lunch at *Mama's Fish House*, a place I discovered the previous year. The legendary eatery is famous for fresh fish and seafood caught early each morning. We were not disappointed. *Mama's* has a knack for making everyone feel like neighbors. We feasted on delectable seafood, and found ourselves chatting with couples from Missouri, Australia, and New Zealand. An afternoon downpour delayed our departure for an hour or so, but the rain only enhanced the vistas of the colorful ocean, palm trees, and cliffs.

Another adventure was just around the corner with our sunset dinner cruise on a 50-foot catamaran. We would meet the yacht at 4:30, so we decided to arrive at 3:00 – just to make sure we were not rushed. We boarded the resort shuttle for the dock in Lahaina at 2:30, and reached our destination in half an hour. The driver assured us we were in the right place and directed us to the dock behind the hotel. We made the trek to the beach as instructed, but soon discovered there was no dock in the area. The temperature was about 85 degrees with no ocean breezes stirring and practically no shade. It was hot. The combination of heat and the half mile hike left me exhausted. Cassandra commandeered a chair from a beachfront bar and planted it in the sand between the hotel property line and the beach. I sat heavily in that chair while she darted off to get some answers. Live bands playing for beachfront cafés for early Happy Hour crowds offered a diversion, but after about 30 minutes or so, I began to wonder. My phone call to Cassandra's cell phone went unanswered. Another half-hour passed before she returned, slightly out of breath. By then I was "well done" and not really interested in her story. For a moment she tried to convince me that I had moved, and my relocation was the reason she couldn't find me. But I gave her *that look*, and she quickly backed off. Apparently she had gotten caught up in the afternoon festivities and became disoriented between beachfront venues. Nevertheless, she managed to find out that in recent weeks the cruise launch point had moved from our current location to the town of Lahaina five miles away. I was livid. I grabbed my cane and hobbled off for the shuttle station. Cassandra followed, imploring me to wait while she tried to call a taxi. I was having none of it. All I wanted was to get back to our suite and cool off. She disappeared once again as I staggered back to the shuttle station. I thought, *She's a big girl. She can find her way back to the suite on her own*. Thirty minutes later, I approached the shuttle station just in time to see the transport slowly roll away, intensifying my agitation. I collapsed in disgust on a bench to catch my breath, fuming over the afternoon's misadventure. But soon I was jolted out of my funk by a blaring taxicab horn. I turned to see Cassandra running toward me from the taxi parked about 100 feet away. "Get your butt in that cab," she ordered as she pointed a perfectly manicured nail toward the idling vehicle. She had spoken to the tour office and confirmed the actual launch point for our voyage. The boat was being held for us.

It took another 10 to 15 minutes to break through the afternoon traffic and reach the dock. As we scrambled to where our ship was supposed to be waiting, we found only an empty slip. The heat was relentless, and I was still exhausted. "I have to sit down," I bayed. With that I planted myself on the concrete steps leading to the pier. Cassandra went off to find a cup of water. In the hubbub I had missed an incoming call from a Captain Caleb of Trilogy Tours. His voicemail indicated that he was looking for us. I was instructed to call him back at an 800 number to arrange a rendezvous. Just as I finished listening to the voicemail, Cassandra returned – without water. Before I launched into my rave, I caught sight of a striking athletic figure as he leapt from a catamaran moored next to the empty slip. He flashed a bright smile and extended his hand toward me. "Are you Mr. Harvey? I'm Captain Turtle." I nodded in the affirmative. Captain Turtle cast his gaze at Cassandra, who somehow was still poised, cool, and looking like a million bucks. She was shaded by a large stylish straw hat and draped in a green and black silk tunic. She seemed to float and flutter like a butterfly. Captain Turtle stuttered slightly, transfixed, as Cassandra sat quietly beside me. The captain continued, "We've been looking for you. Our radios were temporarily out of order and we've been trying to communicate via cell phone." I extended my phone to Captain Turtle and told him that I believed a voicemail I just received from Captain Caleb was for him. I pulled up the message and simultaneously Captain Turtle took out his cell phone and dialed the number he captured from the voicemail. He spoke to Captain Caleb for a few moments and then closed his phone. Still gazing at Cassandra, he extended both his hands toward hers. In return, she placed her hands in his as he raised her to a standing position. I caught a flash of sunlight as it danced off her hazel eyes. "Beautiful lady," the captain cooed, "We can't have you out in this hot sun. Let me take you over to the shade and get you a cold drink of water." With that he escorted Cassandra to a grove of trees about 50 feet away from the dock and encouraged people sitting on a nearby bench to move. Without releasing her hands he provided support while she sat on the vacated bench.

Oh, hell no! How dare they leave me stranded on these hot concrete steps? I pouted. As I began to struggle to my feet, Captain Turtle's Second Mate appeared by my side and escorted me to the bench where Cassandra was perched. "You sit right there. I'll get you some water," the young man said. Captain Turtle was still standing in front of Cassandra, holding her hands in his. "You guys wait here, they're bringing the boat back to port, and I'll help you aboard."

The Second Mate thrust of cup of cold water into my hand, which snapped me back to attention. Had I really witnessed Cassandra casting her spell on yet another total stranger? Admittedly, he was muscular, tall and good-looking. Both of them seemed to be caught in a trance. I thought, *I'm half dead, and these two are doing back strokes in each other's eyes. I don't believe it.* "You wait here. I'll be right back," said the captain, as he sprinted back to his catamaran to continue preparations for his own departure. After about 20 minutes, we heard the rumble of the twin diesel engines as the catamaran artfully backed into the slip. Captain Turtle again leapt from his vessel, and sprinted back to where we were seated. "Your transport has arrived," he said as he took Cassandra's hand once again and led her toward the approaching ship. I hobbled along behind them, taking out my aggression with each tamping of my cane upon the pier. The docking vessel gently came to a halt, and the crew let down the gangway. Captain Turtle escorted Cassandra onto the vessel, as he greeted Captain Caleb. The catamaran was full of guests, each holding a flute of champagne or a glass of wine, staring in disbelief that they had traveled back to the dock to pick up the two of us. The crew greeted us as celebrities. What we did not know is that these cruises *never* return to port to retrieve late arriving guests. The other dinner guests murmured, trying to figure out *who the hell are these people?* Of course, Cassandra was all smiles and warmly greeted everyone as she glided past them on deck. She did look stunning – as freshly pressed as if she had just left the villas. I scoffed with a wry smile, as she worked her magic. A table was waiting mid-ship with our name card, where we were seated and promptly offered wine and champagne. I realized that no one had been served. The other guests had only cocktails or wine. The dinner cruise had waited for *The Harveys* to arrive!

Our catamaran exited the slip and was steered deftly past other vessels meandering in and out of the breakwaters. Smooth jazz wafted across the bow of the yacht as we glided toward the open ocean. The casual and congenial air soon dissolved my dogged annoyance as I fell under the spell of the ocean's smooth and rhythmic motion. Cassandra seemed to sense that I had finally relaxed. She looked at me and winked as if to say, "See, you don't have to control everything. I got this." She turned and drew the table next to her into small talk about Kaho'olawe, the uninhabited island we were now passing as the sun continued its slow descent. For a brief moment clouds hovering above the island threatened showers, but none fell. Sunlight gently pierced the clouds adding a shimmering luster to the view and skipping along the ocean's waves. Salads arrived as our waiter inquired about drinks and condiments. The drama of the previous two hours seemed like someone else's bad dream. Captain Caleb made his way to our table to investigate, I suspected, the mysterious woman who captured the attention of his colleague. He seemed to linger a bit longer at our table, heightening the curiosity of the other guests, as he shared how he acquired the yacht as a young man and abandoned his boring job on the mainland for adventure on the high seas. Captain Caleb was only 36 and had been sailing for ten years. We marveled at his adventurous spirit, throwing caution to the wind to follow his dream. In that moment I was reminded of the words from Bette Midler's song, *The Color of Roses*:

> *It's so hard to touch*
> *What is out of our hands*
> *To know and to trust*
> *What the heart understands.*
>
> *Only the ones who believe*
> *Ever see what they dream*
> *Ever dream what comes true.*

We found ourselves transfixed by yet another brilliant sunset and an evening spent under a fabulous moonlit sky. At the end of our cruise, we returned by taxi to the villas where we were greeted by a young valet whom we had not met. The young man seemed unusually excited as he brought a wheelchair to the taxi, escorting me to the conveyance. Apparently, news that the yacht returned for us had reached the villas already. The young valet chattered incoherently, as I remained in a state of mild euphoria from the cruise, not paying much attention to his babble. Cassandra's pose under the portico invited guests to enter the South lobby lanai. A late evening breeze caused her skirt to dance gracefully. All she needed was her "key light", a camera crew, and frenzied paparazzi. The *diva* was having a moment, but seemed a bit too intrigued by the excitement of the young valet. "I was told you were a big deal back in the day. In what films did you appear in the '80's and '90's? I believe I've seen you in some movie. Give me a title." Initially, I stared vacantly at the young man, but then protested good-naturedly, waving my hands in denial. Admittedly, I was charmed by his naive enthusiasm. As I caught a glimpse of Cassandra, she quickly turned away and pretended to be oblivious to the valet's efforts to identify me. I looked back at the young man and realized the more I protested, the more he was convinced I was trying to remain incognito. I never found out exactly what preposterous story passed her lips, but I suspected the *diva's* flirting with the valets earlier in the week, juxtaposed with the unusual return of the yacht to retrieve us at the pier in Lahaina added to our intrigue as the yet unidentified *It Couple*. Chuckling to myself, I beckoned to Cassandra, and she wheeled me through the lobby back to our Suite. "You know, if you keep up this charade we're going to get evicted and banned from this island."

Our day of departure came all too soon. We packed and made ready for the hours' drive to the Maui airport. Since I was unable to book first-class seats or a direct return flight, our itinerary included a plane change in Honolulu. Remembering the long walk to the departing gate, Cassandra called ahead to reserve a wheelchair, which was waiting at the security checkpoint when we arrived. I was *randomly* selected for a full body search and was escorted to the inspection area, but the security checkpoint line remained in view. Cassandra guarded the wheelchair while the TSA agent patted me down and scanned me for contraband. I have no idea what they were trying to find, but their search seemed clumsy and disorganized. I soon noticed a mild commotion in Cassandra's vicinity and tuned in to hear her exchange with a TSA agent, another beautiful and exotic island man, quickly falling under the *diva's* spell. "I think you need to get in this wheelchair and let me push you around the airport," she cooed in a low sultry voice. "Ma'am, I'll gladly get in that wheelchair and you can push me wherever you want – for as long as you want," the agent replied, gazing into the *diva's* hypnotic eyes.

"Okay. That's it. We're done," I exclaimed to the fumbling TSA agents who had been conducting the search. I grabbed my cane, and hobbled over to the wheelchair and Cassandra, who was breaking her spell on the TSA agent who then slipped away. "We need to get to our gate before you get us arrested for kidnapping a federal employee," I quipped, tapping my cane on the side of the wheelchair. Cassandra sighed, and pushed me slowly toward our gate. "But he was so pretty," she purred. "Yeah – that's what you said about half a dozen other men you've tried to apprehend this week. The TSA should've checked your luggage. I'm sure you have a man or two hidden in there somewhere." We both laughed and proceeded to our gate.

When we arrived she positioned me near the gangway entrance. "Keep your ass in that wheelchair, and don't move. You need to look as pitiful as possible. Drool, if you have to," she ordered. She was determined to elicit special treatment for us. I started to protest and she raised her finger and waved it in my face. "You're not drooling!" Amazingly the ploy worked. About ten minutes later the gate agents arrived and one of them came over and asked for our tickets. "Excuse me, I'll be right back," the agent said. Moments later the agent returned, saying, "I've moved your seating to the first row on the flight to Honolulu. I'm sorry I couldn't put you in the first-class cabin on your flight from Honolulu to Dallas, but the plane is already too full. I'm giving you the best seats available." The agent smiled and went back to her post. Cassandra slapped me gently on the shoulder and winked. "I told you to drool. You should listen to me, Mr. Harvey. I told you before, I got this."

We arrived in Dallas around 5 a.m. on Memorial Day. A friend met us at the airport and drove us to our homes. I rested all day.

The next day at 6 a.m. I showed up at the Advanced Radiology facility for a liver biopsy. Back to reality. The procedure went well. I received the results the following week. On a scale of 1 to 10 (1 being normal and 10 indicating cirrhosis), my results were between 0 and 1. In other words, my liver had not been affected by the hepatitis B, and the antiviral therapy remained highly effective. Tests during my June 13th visit with Dr. Brenner indicated my viral loads were still undetectable. Two days later I met with Dr. Agha for my monthly consult. "I don't know what you've been doing the past month," he said, "but whatever it is, keep doing it. You look *so much better* than you did last month! In May I was a bit concerned with your appearance, but your skin tone is improved and you look great!"

I laughed hysterically inside, taking his reaction as confirmation my clandestine prescription had worked its magic. Someday I may confess my Maui secret to Dr. Agha.

11 My So-Called Love Life

Although my medical trauma has moved me closer to emotional awareness, in truth, I am not an emotionally driven person. My mind thrives on intellection. I seek to understand rather than imagine or emote. I have disciplined myself not to react immediately to what I see or hear. I analyze and contemplate the context before deciding what to make of a situation – whether to take it seriously or whether it was part of some facetious or satirical jest. Only then do I invest verbal comment, intentional action, or feelings. The process may take nanoseconds or several days. While this seems quite natural to me, it seems to puzzle those around me – particularly those who do not know me very well. Years ago, as one of my very best friends and I discussed over dinner the art of flirting – a behavior I never understood – I said with a measure of disdain, "Why don't people just say what they mean? It would save a lot of time and avoid miscommunication." At first she thought I was joking, but when she realized I was dead serious, she quipped, "Reggie, you were cheated as a child. Your box of Cracker Jacks was missing the decoder ring." There was more truth to what she said than she could possibly have imagined.

For years I was somewhat defensive about my intellection, thinking there may be something amiss about the way I was wired, until I read *QUIET: The Power of Introverts in a World That Can't Stop Talking* by Susan Cain (2013). I welcomed Cain's premise that society tends to reward and exalt those who display extroverted characteristics as brilliant thought leaders whose hurried decisiveness tends to be misinterpreted as deep insight and understanding. In fact, these prophets hold very shallow views of the world around them. Cain defines true introverts as those who think deeply about the world they inhabit. She corrects the stereotype that introverts are shy, explaining instead they tend to limit their prolonged exposure to crowds because the white noise of "group think" distracts from the peaceful solitude that catalyzes their pragmatic contemplation. She suggests that without introverts the world would be devoid of the theory of relativity, Chopin's nocturnes, Orwell's *1984* and *Animal Farm, The Cat in the Hat*, Google and *Harry Potter*. No argument from me.

As an introvert, I find peaceful solitude to be indispensable. I am sometimes amazed at the clarity I experience after quiet moments of reflection. I was never very good at meditation, but my free-form method of introspection works quite well. It was during a period of quiet contemplation that I became aware of one of the most poignant revelations of my life's journey: I am emotionally immature. Furthermore, I was able to trace my immaturity to three specific experiences, which occurred early in my life and impacted deeply my understanding and perception of the opposite sex and my social interaction with the world around me. As I have detailed these experiences in prior chapters, I will review them only briefly here.

The first incident occurred when I was seven as I witnessed the scene that played out after my parents learned of my sister's statutory rape and pregnancy. I could not reconcile what I saw in that moment with any part of our family's life, but the extraordinary actions of those present – my dad and Mr. Treadwell wrestling on the floor, Sandra crying uncontrollably, my mom standing aside, detached, as if in another world – signaled to my seven-year-old brain that *something* was drastically wrong. Although I could not comprehend the drama unfolding before my eyes, today I feel certain that I was emotionally scarred by what I witnessed and by living through the this assault visited not only upon my sister, but on my entire family. We never discussed the horror, hurt, and anguish, even though it was surely a public secret. We did not undergo therapy. This experience was one of the first cracks in the once fine vase. With no one to interpret this event for me, I was left to process it on my own, as I grew older, and to piece together my perception, bit by bit.

Owing to the deep social divide in Waterloo's African-American community, I did not have normal social interactions with children my age. Nearly all of the black residents were former sharecroppers from Mississippi, or their direct descendants, i.e., they were blue collar workers with limited education. Although they respected my parents, they did not know exactly what to think of this highly educated couple. There may have been an element of fear involved. They kept their distance. As a result, I did not have friends. I did not have birthday parties, because no one would come. I never experienced puppy love or a teenage crush. Having missed out on the usual interactions with girls, my only context for sex was what happened to my sister. By the time I was a teenager, I was imprinted with my own set of warped beliefs about sex. In my immature mind, sex *was* rape. Clearly, the rapist was a social predator. I never wanted anyone to think I could harm them as this rapist had harmed my sister. I did not want to be a rapist. In my mind, sex must be feared first and foremost. Sexual arousal could be life-threatening. And sex was a terrible weapon used to inflict infinite pain on unsuspecting people. Therefore, I made myself emotionally, socially, and sexually unavailable, hoping to prevent ever being perceived as a rapist. This was not logical. This was fear. For many, many years it was not even a *conscious* fear—I did not realize I harbored this fear until I was in my 40's.

The second incident occurred when I was 15. The isolation I felt growing up in Iowa was temporarily quelled when I met a boy whose life paralleled my own in many ways. Particularly, we both felt keenly the social pressures placed on us because our demanding fathers were prominent and influential men. He was as estranged from his father as I was from mine. We became pen pals, sharing in our correspondence these deeply personal feelings about our lives. My friend's father, a state senator, showed up at our home one Saturday afternoon with him in tow, and an intercepted letter in his hand. Subsequently, I was ordered by my father to cease and desist from this correspondence, which from my perspective was beneficial, enjoyable and entirely innocent. I was completely confused. I had done something wrong, but I did not know what. With no explanation from my father, my teenage mind could only conclude that divulging emotional feelings with another person was as sinister and damaging as sexual desire. I was too naïve and socially inept to connect emotional and sexual expression, but I felt certain there was something dark and sinister surrounding both. Not wanting to experience my father's extreme displeasure, my solution once again was avoidance. My pathological design was simply to avoid sharing my emotions with another person. It would be several decades before I could surmise that my father and the senator erroneously interpreted the correspondence with my pen pal to represent a foray into a gay relationship.

The third major contributor to my emotional immaturity occurred during my senior year in high school when a girl I had never met claimed I dated, "pinned", and then dumped her during the preceding summer. Her malicious fabrication came close to ruining my entire senior year. Observing her effective manipulation of students, teachers, and administrators made me forever suspicious of hidden agendas. I was disgusted, angry, and hurt, especially with my teachers and other adults for believing this girl. Seeing how a female could cause the entire school to impugn my character and censure my treatment of the opposite sex – without a shred of evidence – virtually dashed any hope I may have held of establishing a close relationship with the opposite sex. I regarded females as untrustworthy, manipulative, insincere, and morally reprehensible. Although I did not discuss these thoughts with anyone, I was careful to I avoid being used in that way ever again.

My strategy of avoidance is key. I decided on a collection of attitudes, beliefs, and codes of behavior – taboos, if you will – designed to insulate me from the extreme pain I associated with these experiences. The problem is my taboos were rooted in faulty premises, contributing in no positive way to my mental or emotional development.

Given all this, it is not surprising I have been unsuccessful at finding romance. Truthfully, "finding romance" is a poor way to describe the quest for lasting companionship. When Dr. Agha entered my hospital room, I am sure he believed the patient before him was a promiscuous, drug-using gay man. He was mistaken.

I can't say that my failure to find a life partner is surprising. Here, again, my emotional immaturity resulting from illogical taboos has come into play. Another contributing factor was growing up in a community that was intellectually sterile. The cocoon in which my family insulated itself resulted in further isolation. With few social outlets, I occupied myself with academic pursuits, adventures in literature, travel, and the arts. People around me often made assumptions and inferences about my so-called love life. I have grown accustomed to their disbelief that my life experience is virtually blank in that area; that I prefer to be alone. I have tried to distinguish between the choice to be alone and the state of loneliness, but my words seem to fall on deaf ears. People presume I am hiding lascivious and salacious secrets, or I am simply lying about my celibacy. I am not saying that I have lived the past 46 years entirely without sex. What I *am* saying is those experiences have been infrequent, clumsily discovered, and ineptly accomplished.

For many people, the weekend is party time – a chance to take part in the flirting and dating rituals that are fodder for TV commercials. That has never been my world. I am not complaining about it, I am simply establishing that such exploits are not part of my experience. Perhaps a survey of my weekends in solitude will provide a tangible frame of reference. Between 1980 and 2016, I have spent about 70% of my weekends alone. So the cumulative amount of weekend-time I have not been involved in some scheduled activity or recreational adventure during this period would translate into 62,880 hours, 2,620 days, 1310 weekends or roughly seven years. Understand, that I am not whining. I am highlighting only that my weekends have not been met with great anticipation. I accepted what I had to look forward to most often: *nothing*.

I feel it must be said that I am happy with my male identity. I have no issues with gender confusion. What baffles many is that I find most people (women as well as men) to be physically unattractive and uninteresting. For example, I never understood the fascination men seem to have with women's breasts – every human being has a pair. Although women's breasts are often more prominent, most are not particularly attractive or well cared for. Oprah devoted entire shows to drive home the point that the majority of women don't know how to select the appropriately sized bra to provide "the girls" with adequate comfort and support. Regardless of the bra issue, I simply do not appreciate the connection between sexual attraction and breasts. Again, everybody has a pair. In general, I find most women fail to present themselves in a manner that accentuates their physical assets. I agree that beauty is not necessarily linked to a particular body type or set of features. For me, women who are stunning (regardless of age) have discovered a combination of physical fitness, posture, natural grace and a sense of how to dress appropriately for their body type.

Then there is the issue of makeup. I swear, some women must use a trowel to apply it. They wear too much or they wear the wrong tone, resulting in a garish and unflattering appearance. I can only surmise there simply must be a discrepancy between what they see in the mirror and how they appear to others. It is not necessary to apply all that goop. Attempting to mimic models on the cover of fashion magazines is an exercise in futility. Cindi Crawford has admitted that even *she* does not look like the Cindi Crawford we see in her magazine photos. She says models are wrapped in electrician's tape and saran wrap and the fashions are pinned and sewn to fit their figure. The lights are set just right as makeup artists and hair stylists spend hours attaining a particular "look." Even after hours of wrapping, pinning and sewing, the photos that finally make it to magazine covers (or the articles within) are usually airbrushed to further perfect the image. It is impossible for any *real* person to achieve "the look."

I have spent way too many words on this, so let me say even the few who stick out in the crowd do not evoke sexual desire on my part. The whole "natural attraction" thing does not work for me. What I do find attractive is a person's personality, wit, talent, attitude, and human kindness. When that is properly packaged I am intrigued beyond words. Thus the pool from which I could select a mate is virtually dry. Perhaps this is why I find those people boring or off-putting in some manner whom so many of my friends have introduced to me, in their desperate matchmaking attempts. My friends swoon in anguish that I am alone, not understanding their choices are based upon criteria intriguing only to them. I know they mean well, and I appreciate their effort, but I wish they would cease and desist.

With that off my chest, I surrender my soapbox, and move on to a more substantive point: the impact of my emotional immaturity and psychological distress upon my so-called love life. I want to be entirely transparent here about my infrequent and unsuccessful attempts to normalize for myself the game of "hooking up."

In 1979 at age 24, I accepted a position with Dow Chemical USA and settled in Clear Lake City, a suburb of Houston. With a metropolitan area rivaling the geographic footprint of Los Angeles, Houston was a modern version of the *Wild, Wild West*. The suburb of Katy was a 2 ½ hour freeway drive from Galveston in rush-hour traffic. At one inch below sea level, Houston's network of bayous is intended to provide flood protection. The George Bush International Airport was a 52-mile drive north-northwest from my home in Clear Lake. I could see the National Aeronautics and Space Administration (NASA) headquarters across the vacant field from my front door.

Houston was home to 1.6 million people in 1980, a population 21 times that of Waterloo, Iowa. The scale of Houston offered vast opportunities for exploration, which I embraced with open arms. I was excited to embark on my career. The inconveniences of a large city are counterbalanced by the diversity of cultures, services and neighborhoods. My work schedule required me to rise no later than 4:30 a.m. to carpool to Dow Chemical, 70 miles south-southwest of Clear Lake. Yes, I did say "carpool." Dow Chemical employed more than 25,000 people at the Texas location, and 700 of us carpooled daily from various parts of Houston. During my first six months on the job, I maintained my 4:30 a.m. wake-up schedule on weekends, striking out to explore new destinations for food, goods, and services throughout the metropolitan area. It was wise to be on the road by 5:30 a.m. to start errands, because travel to just about any destination required 30 to 60 minutes. I would map out my routes and spend the next six to eight hours running my errands. As a recent college graduate, I needed just about everything for my new home.

One Saturday while running errands, I stopped for lunch at a nondescript restaurant in a small strip mall near downtown Houston. During my meal I noticed a gentleman across the room who wore overalls with the PEPSI logo. He stared at me and did not look away, even when I caught him staring. I thought he must be attracted to me in some way, because he didn't know me and there was no other explanation for his behavior. I found people of Houston to be very forward – there were no strangers. I left money on the table to cover my meal and returned to my car. The PEPSI guy followed me outside at a distance and walked towards his delivery truck. As I pulled off the parking lot, the PEPSI truck followed in casual pursuit. I dismissed it, at first, as coincidence. Ten minutes later I noticed in my rearview mirror what I thought was a different PEPSI delivery truck. As I drove, I made plans to unload the car and install the goods I purchased that morning. I exited the freeway for Clear Lake City as the PEPSI van followed. Intrigued, I drove to my condo on Bay Area Blvd, and parked. To my surprise the *PEPSI* van parked across the street. I got out of my car and was met by a pleasant voice, "Hi. I wanted to introduce myself in the restaurant, but you seemed to be on a mission. My name is Mike. I drive all over Houston restocking vending machines and convenience stores, but I've never been out here. Is that the Johnson Space Center across the way?" I was at a loss for words, but I managed to reply, "Yes, that's NASA headquarters." "Wow, so that's where the magic happens," Mike exclaimed quietly as he stared at the space center's administration building. "I've got to head home in a couple hours, but I'm a little beat from being on the road since 2 a.m.. Do you mind if we sit and chat for a while? I've got an extra six pack of soda I'd be willing to share." My curiosity was on overload. Mike looked like your average southern good-old boy. I watched him reach into the back of the truck and pull out a six pack. He held up the cans for me to see as he closed the back of the truck. "OK," I replied, "as long as you help me unload my car." "No problem," Mike answered. I had already opened my trunk for unloading, but Mike handed me the cans of soda. "You go on up and I'll bring these things for you." I went up the stairs, unlocked the door, and headed for the kitchen to get glasses and ice. I returned to my living room to find Mike placing the items from my trunk neatly on the landing at my front door. He left the door open as if to ask permission to enter. I nodded, indicating a side chair. I handed him a glass full of ice and a can of soda. I shut the door and we sat and talked – Mike in the side chair and me on the sofa – for about a half an hour. He told me about his two kids, and shared a few war stories about his adventures delivering beverages around the city. He was polite, athletically built, and was a devoted fan of the Houston Astros. His conversation remained light and upbeat. He downed the soda and asked for another. I pointed to the kitchen, telling him they were on the counter. He returned with two cans, one tucked under his arm and the other he opened and poured into my empty glass. He picked up his glass on the floor next to the side chair, and moved to the opposite end of the sofa. After refilling his class he fell silent and stared at me for a while. He drained his glass, set it on the coffee table, reached over and took my glass out of my hands and set it on the table. I was uncertain why he did this, until while retrieving my glass he held onto my hand and pulled me toward him on the sofa. Before I knew it he kissed me and held me tightly. My curiosity got the best of me. I didn't fight him off because his movements were so certain and definite. What perplexed me most was he seemed to be a typical guy's guy. He had just been sharing stories about his kids and baseball, but now he held me firmly in his embrace. Mike rested his cheek against mine and continued to hold me and gently, slowly rocking back and forth. He then pulled away slightly while gently holding both my shoulders. "I want you to take me. Make love to me." That was all he said. I wasn't certain what he meant or what he wanted me to do. He seemed to understand I was at a loss, so he coached me through what he wanted. He removed his clothes and positioned himself in front of me. Without further comment he guided me inside him.

I had never had sex with anyone, and I was 24 years old. When it was over he stood up and went to the bathroom. He quickly returned with a warm wet washcloth, and handed it to me. I cleaned myself and adjusted my clothing. By the time I finished he was back in his uniform, and seated once again in the side chair. My head was reeling as I replayed the scene in my head. No words had been spoken for five minutes or so. I wanted to ask why he had wanted *this* to happen, but I couldn't figure out how to put the words together to form a coherent sentence. Mike began to speak calmly while looking me directly in the eyes. "From time to time I get tired of being the strong one, and I just need someone else – a man – to make me feel it's OK to exhale." I could see that he understood I was still confused, but mesmerized. "I saw you at lunch, and you seemed to be a cool cat. So I followed you in the hopes that you would be that man for me." Before I could speak, Mike made one last comment. "I make deliveries at that strip mall every other week, and have lunch at that restaurant. I'd like to see you again. If you show up, that would be great. If not take care of yourself." With that he left, closing the door behind him. I could hear him on the stairway. But I couldn't move. I sat there in a state of shock until I heard his truck pull away. Then I remembered my things stacked on the landing outside. I got up and retrieved them and continued with my original plan to install the items in my home. I never told anyone about what had happened. But I played the scene over and over in my head. What I could not resolve was how confident, but gentle Mike had been. He seemed to be aware of my immaturity, but he told me he had hoped I "...would be that man..." for him.

Over the next six weeks, I returned to that strip mall and found him twice. Each time we repeated the ritual, and I began to accept that he wanted this to happen. This was my first sexual encounter and I was intrigued by it all. I didn't even know how to have sex. It was like an out-of-body experience. When it happened a second time, I thought, *is this really happening? Is this how it is supposed to be?* I never expected my first sexual encounter to be with a man. Still, I didn't question my gender identity. Although it was not a "relationship", this human being desired me for some reason. I did not know this was even possible. I got caught up in the physical desire that was playing itself out.

During the next six months or so, I did not see Mike. There was too much going on. I began to travel with my work. Houston experienced two 100-year floods. The first occurred in June. I had never experienced torrential rains like that. Two tropical storms stalled in the Gulf of Mexico and continued to dump rain on the city. It rained constantly for a week before the apex of the deluge, and on the day of the tipping point, the downpour relentlessly pelted an area over 100 miles wide. Clear Lake rose 12 feet in 24 hours. Everything was flooded by at least 4 feet of water. By September, most flood victims had made significant progress toward re-establishing a sense of normalcy, when a second 100-year flood swept through Houston. Water backed up through the 54-mile Ship Channel and spilled over into the bayous crisscrossing the city.

In October, I found tucked in my doorframe a note from Mike with his pager number. I called the number and received a call back. Mike let me know his delivery routes had been redrawn several times due to the summer storms. We made arrangements to rendezvous. This time, Mike confirmed his devotion to his marriage and to his kids, and attempted to explain again his desire for occasional male "companionship." He seemed almost near tears as he shared the angst surrounding his compulsion. I was confused. I did not expect this otherwise macho man to become so emotional. And if he was so committed to his family, what the hell was I in the picture for?

That was the last time I saw Mike.

The experience raised more questions than answers. Having grown up entertaining myself and interacting with adults 30 years or more my senior, I was accustomed to being alone. In Houston, I engaged in shared activities with people – excursions, dinner and such – but these settings were about the activity; there was nothing personal. I enjoyed knowing people professionally and the comradery of finding our way in our careers, but these were only associates. There was no one I considered a friend. My focus was on intellectual pursuits, solving problems for my employer. I worked. And I had no sexual fantasies. Sex with Mike was not something I was looking for or something I encouraged. I did not judge it. There was no preference on my part. It was just an experience.

It would be another four years before my next sexual encounter.

By 1983 I was one year into my transition from Houston's petrochemical industry to real-time weapon systems software development for the DoD in Dallas. I found outlets for my musical interests. At the University of Iowa and UT Austin I had sung in collegiate chorales. In Houston I had been a member of a semi-professional madrigal group, The Nova Singers. I was also a paid singer in the chancel choir of First Presbyterian Houston, a megachurch with about 3,500 members. My performances in Dallas were wider in scope, including R&B, jazz, and classical oratorio. Performing with celebrated pianist, Fred Crane, I won the 1983 jazz showcase at Tim Ballard's. That win resulted in a week-long stay in Los Angeles where I presented my demo tape to the American Song Festival ASF talent committee.

On the eve of my departure from LA, I found myself at an all-night diner near Sunset Boulevard. There were not many patrons so after my meal I decided to linger over several cups of coffee. When a man at an adjacent table asked me to pass a condiment to him that was missing from his table, we struck up a casual conversation, with him doing most of the talking. His personality and manner were engaging. After about 20 minutes, he moved to my table and our discussion continued. It felt as though we had known each other all our lives.

For a moment I thought of Beverly, a psychology professor who had been my neighbor in Clear Lake City. She told me that such a sense of long-term familiarity with a stranger could be attributed to "a shared dictionary." When a stranger phrases responses in nearly the same way you would, or expresses the same fleeting observations you would make, the brain recognizes the speech patterns and sentiments. Thus there is a perceived familiarity.

Four hours later I was still drinking coffee and eating pie and talking to Tony, a professional baseball umpire. I finally told him I had to catch a plane in the morning and needed to get some sleep. He thanked me for the rich conversation, and we exchanged phone numbers. As we stood to leave, I could see that he was about six feet four with an extremely muscular build. The stocky jock type that would have stuffed me in a locker had we met in high school. We approached the exit and Tony turned toward me, flashing a broad smile. For the first time I noticed he was very fine-looking – quite exotic. His face was broad with a square jaw and there was a subtle cleft in his chin. He looked like a leading man in a 1940's film noir. His slightly swarthy complexion glowed. I couldn't believe this strong and charismatic person spent nearly five hours talking attentively to me. The next day I returned to Dallas and submerged myself in work, never expecting to hear from Tony again.

Contrary to my assumptions, Tony called me every evening. He had a fabulous sense of humor, and was always poking fun at baseball (his favorite sport, naturally), politics, and society in general. Our calls usually lasted an hour or two during the week and longer on weekends. We enjoyed our talks, and they never covered the same territory. My long distance phone bills shot up to several hundred dollars, so I could not imagine how much he invested in "Ma Bell", as he did most of the calling. In those days there were no free long distance calling plans. Tony was making a sizeable investment in getting to know me. I surmised he pulled in an income equal to or greater than my own. Tony became my social outlet. I continued my volunteer work with the Dallas Office of Cultural Affairs and my performances, but my talks with Tony were personal, adventurous, and fun. His frequent and lengthy calls eventually made me realize the depth of his connection with me. His interest in my career and in my view of the world was endearing. No one made me feel that way since my days at Miss Tread's dining room table or around the Christmas tree at Granny's farmhouse. He was not family – he was still practically a stranger – but he had the amazing ability to break through my walls and *speak* to me. Somehow I knew he meant no harm to me. Everything about him challenged the illusory taboos I held on to as a means of self-defense.

At Tony's urging, I made arrangements to return to Los Angeles and spend a week with him.

Labor Day weekend I headed west in my new Isuzu Impulse, a small, sporty 3-door lift-back coupe, introduced in the U.S. that year. It was exhilarating to put my fuel-efficient sports car through its paces on the open highway, and to anticipate exploring a budding friendship.

Passing through El Paso meant I had put 800 miles between me and the safety of my home. I could see the twinkling lights of Texas in my rear view mirror and Mexico to the south against a completely blackened night sky. There was no turning back now. I was committed to completing the trip.

Tony was athletic and handsome and I was intrigued by him. Perhaps, this trip would be my chance to discover why. Our conversations had been about all kinds of things – life. I knew he had an interest in me as a person. My limited social intelligence offered no answers. But this could be my chance to experience an interaction consciously – to see how things unfolded before my watchful eyes. I could come up with and ask questions to help me understand how this was supposed to work. This was all in my head and had nothing to do with my heart.

I drove all night. I made the 1600 mile drive in two days. As the sun rose gently behind me I realized spending time with Tony would be similar to mailing my next letter to my pen pal from twelve years ago, but better. I would have the chance to sit face-to-face and asked the questions I had been too naïve to probe as a teenager. A momentary pang of uneasiness swept through me, but was washed away with the serenely persistent rising of the sun.

Around noon Saturday I pulled up to Tony's East L.A. residence and parked. I went up to his door and knocked tentatively. The door opened to a face that seemed at first unfamiliar. For a brief second I panicked, thinking I must be at the wrong house. But before I could gather my thoughts, I was physically trapped in a bear hug and lifted into the air. "You made it! Man, it's good to see you. Come in, come in!" the man exclaimed as he lowered me to the floor. I was frozen. The man kept talking rapidly and excitedly, picking up my bags and gently shoving me into his living room. I don't remember what he said, but I sat down clumsily, staring. Slowly the familiar voice confirmed that this massively framed figure was Tony. It was like seeing an avatar with the blended features of Clint Walker (star of *Cheyenne*, a popular TV western series from 1955 to 1963) and Tom Selleck. And then there was that smile that was as broad as the horizon. This person was truly excited that I had actually made the trip. I could not process anyone being that happy see me. It was overwhelming.

Everything he did from that moment on was intended to ensure that I felt special and had fun. Unbeknownst to Tony, *fun* was not a familiar objective for me. Certainly, I enjoyed my intellectual and academic pursuits, but I could not reliably plan or schedule *fun*. Tony's life was different. He enthusiastically outlined the weekend itinerary, assuring me that I need not worry about anything.

That same evening we took my car to a posh restaurant in West Hollywood, Le Cage aux Folles. We were seated European-style at a table with three other (heterosexual, middle-aged) couples whom we did not know. The meal was exquisite, and the environment was reminiscent of elegant supper clubs from the 40's and 50's. I felt as though I was in a movie from that era, especially when a waiter ushered in Lana Turner, the president of NBC television, and an MGM movie producer and seated them at an adjacent table. Tony seemed glad to introduce me to everyone, and no one we encountered seemed the least bit offended that we were together. Looking back, I was probably the only one who was slightly uncomfortable, but my discomfort was overshadowed by the sheer awe of being wined and dined. After a brilliant musical floor show, we left the restaurant and Tony drove us to Circus-Circus, a West Coast version of New York's *Studio 54*. *Circus-Circus* was a sprawling disco, spinning music that was off the chain – Prince, Stevie Wonder, Average White Band, Pointer Sisters, Patti LaBelle, Barbra Streisand, Gladys Knight, Earth Wind and Fire, David Bowie – and of course, Michael Jackson. When the valets opened the car doors and Tony got out, a special excitement seemed to take over the people waiting in line. The bouncers eagerly waved Tony and me to the front of the line and affectionately slapped Tony on the back as we entered this fantasyland. It was 1983, and everyone dressed in their finest fashions to party down. Grace Jones may have been a celebrity in New York and Europe, but Tony was her male counterpart in Hollywood. Every now and then my computerized brain would process the conundrum that a major league baseball umpire, a massive athlete – who could dance his ass off – was proud to be seen with me. The only component of this fantasy that did not seem to fit was me.

Everyone in Circus-Circus seemed to know Tony or wanted to be photographed with him. People were ecstatic to be acknowledged with a wave of his hand or to hear him shout their name and greet them personally. When someone approached him, however casually or intentionally, he never missed an opportunity to grab hold of my shoulder or arm, pulling me next to him to introduce me. Although some were curious, having never seen me before, they quickly welcomed me as if to comply with some unwritten protocol. Throughout the evening I was bewildered by how happy Tony was to be in my company. He was so comfortable with me that I was forced to let down my guard and just have fun. I accepted he was my escort, my bodyguard, and my devotee. No one dared offend me or make me feel uncomfortable – and no one wanted to. I felt completely safe and, dare I say, "normal" in public for the first time. I was not preoccupied with fitting in and I was not on the sidelines as a mere spectator – I was center stage and everybody accepted that I belonged there. There was nothing weird about me.

And that was just Saturday night. We spent the next five days zipping around Orange County. At every venue – the shipyards, the farmers market, sports and training facilities, restaurants or Marina del Rey – Tony presented me as his best friend. I didn't get it at the time, but while Tony was a joyful extrovert in public, he was really quite lonely. In his public persona, he was the rock of Gibraltar and the life of the party. Through our daily conversations, he decided I was someone he could trust with his demons and innermost frailties. We talked as if we had grown up together.

Thursday was my last day in L.A. before hitting the road back to Dallas. Upon returning from the day's adventures, we entered Tony's house to find his childhood friend, Louisa, preparing dinner. I learned that evening that Louisa was escaping an abusive marriage. I found her to be very kind. That weekend, her two young children were staying with her mother. At five feet five inches and about 135 pounds, she carried a few extra pounds, but retained a nice figure and appeared to take good care of herself. Dinner was scrumptious, capped off with one of the best carrot cakes I have ever eaten. Tony helped clear the table, but neither allowed me to assist.

The three of us fell into a very natural conversation, during which I learned Louisa's backstory. In the middle of arranging for my fun and fantasy, Tony had been arranging living accommodations for Louisa as she formalized her separation and future divorce. Evidently, the courts had already served Louisa's estranged husband with a temporary restraining order (TRO), giving her a chance to exhale from her waking nightmare. Although Tony and Louisa had been playmates as toddlers, and became "besties" through elementary and middle school, Tony only met Louisa's future husband during high school. He was afraid of Tony, and early on, kept his interests in Louisa subdued. That is, he lurked in the shadows of her circle of care until Tony was inducted into military service in the late 1960's and deployed to Vietnam, joining the faceless marionettes caught up in the fog of war.

With Tony out of the picture, Louisa's future husband wooed her, convincing her to marry. Their first several years were peppered with the kind of spats known to many newlyweds. Louisa never developed with him the type of nurturing and protective bond she and Tony shared. After the birth of their first child, the spats escalated rapidly to verbal, and then physical abuse. By the time their second child was born, Louisa was routinely subjected to beatings, and being locked out of the house. She became a punching bag, dissipating whatever seemed at the moment to anger her husband. When Tony returned to LA, he discovered his "bestie" was in hiding, and her children were being shuttled among extended family. For me, the story timeline is a bit jumbled, but I surmised the TRO had been issued fairly recently. I learned Louisa would be staying with Tony until her new living arrangements could be finalized. He could guarantee her safety until court protections were put in motion, and she could "disappear." More carrot cake and pots of coffee saw us late into the night. At about 11:30 we all said good night and retired for the evening.

I had been sleeping with Tony in his bed the entire trip, but we had not engaged in anything sexual. We usually lay in bed musing over the future, finding comfort at being able to discuss openly our uncertainties about life. It was like a continuation of our long-distance phone calls. Before dozing off, Tony would wrap me in his muscular arms and pull me close to his chest. I had not been held like that by another human being since I was four or five years old, certainly never in my adult life. It was a new experience, yet there was a familiarity about it – feeling the heat of his body against mine, and the rhythmic rise and fall of his immense chest as he breathed. Sometimes I would fall asleep within minutes. Other nights I would relax in his arms listening to him breathe until he fell asleep, as I found myself becoming attached to this living teddy bear. The potential for emotion entered my head from somewhere, and I found myself wondering how Tony *felt* about me. This was entirely new. I was not accustomed to wondering about how anyone *felt* about me. Life for me was like a chemical experiment – a system to be analyzed. Reagents, time, temperature, and pressure were elements that forced a reaction to take place with predictable results. Elements could be manipulated for a certain outcome. Of course, in this system there was no room for emotion.

That Thursday evening, Tony quietly got out of the bed and disappeared for a few minutes. He returned and climbed back under the covers. I was in my usual stupor until I felt someone else lie down beside me. It was Louisa. I opened my eyes and started to get up, until I felt Tony's substantial hand on my shoulder gently reassuring me I had no reason to flee. No words were exchanged. The heat of Tony's body was intoxicating, as was the pine forest musk of his scent. Louisa smelled of freshly cut roses as she gently pulled me toward her. Her silky mane of hair caressed my shoulders and her confidence encouraged me to offer no resistance. I don't know if it was the anticipation that Tony might make love to me that last night or the shock of this new experience with a woman's intimate invitation, but suddenly I felt her hand confidently guiding me inside her body. She held me firmly and rubbed her cheek against mine as she undulated gently in rhythm to Tony's audible breathing. He did not join in, but lay there gently caressing my back. I understood what was happening, and I was not repulsed in any way. Interestingly, I could not distinguish between the extent to which I was physically aroused and the calculations taking place in my head. I recalled Louisa's tragic story told over cups of coffee and carrot cake a few hours earlier and I was keenly aware that this was likely the first time in a very long while that she had been able to feel safe, enjoying gentle lovemaking without the fear of being beaten or raped by a man who was supposed to cherish her. Somehow these realizations posited empathy for Louisa, as I compared her present enjoyment with intercourse to the emptiness I imagined my sister felt during her assault. This was the flip side of the same coin; no abuse was taking place. Could it be possible to offer a woman comfort through the act of sexual desire? For more than two decades I believed this to be impossible. While contemplating these new possibilities, I became conscious that Louisa was lying still. I had not achieved an orgasm but I did feel a psychological release. Tony continued gently stroking my back. After a few minutes of quiet, Louisa gathered her robe and left the room. Tony went to the bathroom and returned with a hot damp cloth. Pulling back the bed covers he very gently washed me, and tossed the wash cloth on the floor. He turned me to face him and moved himself close to me, placing his large hand behind my head, guiding my face against his chest. He kissed me softly several times, and ran his hand down the middle of my lower back. With that he fell asleep, with the rhythmic breathing I had come to know by now. I immediately fell fast asleep.

The next morning we were awakened by the warm radiance of the serenely persistent sun falling through the Venetian blinds. Tony asked if I slept well, and I assured him that I had. We both showered and dressed and entered the dining room to find food already on the table accompanied by freshly squeezed orange juice and hot coffee. There was no tension among us during our three-way breakfast conversation. After eating I packed the rest of my things and made ready for my road trip home. Just before noon, I said goodbye to Louisa. Tony walked me to my car, carrying my bag and placing it in the hatchback. Before I could open the car door he gathered me one last time in that vice-like, teddy bear embrace in which it is almost impossible to breathe, and kissed me. He opened the door for me and I climbed in. As I slowly pulled away from the curb he stood there in the street, having held me in the light of day for all his neighbors to see, and lifted those massive arms, waving them back and forth above his head. In my rearview mirror, I could see him continuing to wave until I lost sight of him as I turned the corner. I had a lot to think about during the next 1600 miles.

I was mentally and emotionally numb during much of the return trip. I grappled with the confirmed affection that Tony had demonstrated towards me. But every time I swooned with that lighter-than-air feeling, I would crash to the ground with the weight of Tony's devotion to Louisa. I vaguely recall that somewhere during the previous night's dinner there had been discussions of marriage between Louisa and Tony. If that was part of Tony's plan to bring stability to Louisa and her kids, then where was there room for Tony and me? Wait. What did I think "Tony and me" meant? There was no "Tony and me" … was there? I would drive for hours – distracted by music blasting from the car stereo. When a tape ran out, or the radio fell silent in a dead broadcast zone, my emotional conundrum would come roaring back between my ears. What could possibly explain the duality of Tony's commitment to marry his "bestie" to protect her and the children, and his overt physical and spiritual pursuit of my affection?

The following week Tony resumed his phone calls, updating me on some of his friends and associates I met during my visit. Mostly, I listened to his adventures, saying very little about my own. I listened trying still to understand my place in his life. I was confused about why he was so happy to be seen with me and so eager to introduce me to people, since he was such an attractive presence whose attention people coveted. I knew he was a real person now, but I was so overwhelmed by the way he treated me – the pedestal he put me on – that I failed to ask the questions I needed answered. I left L.A. no wiser about relationships in general and no more clarity about our interactions than I had been before the trip. This was a serious mistake on my part.

After a few weeks I mentioned that I was thinking about returning to school to get a degree in computer science, a relatively new field at the time. I shared with Tony that my experience working in weapon systems software engineering for DoD may give me an advantage in pursuing this course of study. To my surprise Tony asked if I would consider enrolling at a school in Southern California: UCLA, Cal State, Pepperdine, California Polytech, or University of San Diego, to name a few. He told me I could live with him. I was shocked that he was so eager for me to return, but I believed his offer to be a sincere one. I told him I would think about it.

The next week Tony called me as excited as he had been to see me at his front door. He had been selected to umpire the baseball competitions at the 1984 Olympic Games in Los Angeles. He would have access to special passes, and wanted to confirm that I would come to L.A. for the Olympics. He also asked whether I was any closer to making a decision about enrolling at a college in Orange County. I began to think he was serious about building a life with me, but as I saw it, we were not having a romance. And perhaps I was a bit insecure about the idea of competing with his fan base. What I did not "see" was the sincerity of his connection with me, and the comfort I offered him by just being me. In that moment I rejected the notion that I would uproot my life and relocate across country. I communicated firmly and emphatically that I did not believe we should continue this banter – no matter how intoxicating it may be. Upon hearing my words, Tony fell silent. With that, our interpersonal adventure came to an abrupt end.

Tony was 5 to 10 years older than I, which may have accounted for a difference in our perspectives and understanding of life. The silliness of my argument (which is clear as I write this) is that I really did not have a life in Dallas. Sure, I did things. I worked at my day job, I performed, I volunteered for advisory boards in the performing arts community, but I was not really living. My busy-ness allowed me to avoid questioning the strictures of my taboos. I performed occasionally in recitals and oratorios, which culminated with my portrayal of two tenor roles (as Ned, the conjurer, and Andy, Treemonisha's good friend) in Scott Joplin's opera *Treemonisha* presented by the Dallas Symphony in 1986. That performance to a sold-out audience of season ticket holders received favorable reviews in *The Dallas Morning News*. However, interpreting these two roles conjured my emotional angst regarding friendship and personal relationships. That would be my last public performance.

I never heard from Tony again. I wonder occasionally how different my life would be if I had summoned the courage to make a different choice. In the ensuing decades I came to understand the fault lines I was unwilling to cross in 1983. Tony was an extrovert. I am an introvert. How would that work? Love was a fault line. The idea that I could have a romantic experience was an untested hypothesis. I thought nobody wanted me, but he did. Homosexuality was a fault line. I was a man and he was a man. I was not sure how they felt about that in L.A., but I was uncomfortable with it. I was unavailable to anyone, but he risked wanting me and having me in his life anyway. All of these were fault lines for me. Truthfully, I would probably have fucked up his life, because I was so afraid to expose myself emotionally to anyone. I would eventually come to accept the authenticity of Tony's feelings. I have regretted the choice I made for over 30 years.

It occurred to me that that Tony was one of the "sad young men" whom Roberta Flack sang about so mournfully in *The Ballad of Sad Young Men*. Perhaps that explained it. Tony blamed himself for not being available for his childhood "bestie" in her time of need. He had failed to protect someone he dearly loved while abducted to a napalm-ridden jungle some 7,600 miles away. It became his mission to never abandon anyone again – thus the effusive role he played in the Circus-Circus community. His new assignment was also therapy for the suppressed guilt he felt. The guilt of abandonment. He took on the role of providing solace to all within his circle of care. Wow ... how had I not seen it before? And the familiarity (that shared non-verbal dictionary) I sensed during the marathon conversation in that Sunset Boulevard diner was predicated on the unresolved trauma attaching us both to Vietnam. Though we never discussed the war, we were both "sad young men", with vastly different circumstances leading us to the same pseudo persona. I suspect I was able somehow to provide Tony a safe place to exhale. Could our mutual attraction have been rooted in our disparate, unresolved angst over the Vietnam War? The same war that felled a generation like a chain saw fells trees in the forest?

I have never received another offer like Tony's. I did not know such an offer was even possible. To this day, whenever I enjoy a moist, flavorful serving of my favorite dessert – carrot cake – I am flooded with a waterfall of memories.

Growth is always a positive outcome, but it can be so damn painful.

In 2001 at age 46, I transitioned from 15 years' employment with aerospace companies, and was firmly entrenched in logistics software system integration. After leaving DoD I was invited to work for a rising boutique technical engineering firm in Silicon Valley. I later became director of enterprise solutions for British/U.S. enterprise. While on assignment in Great Britain, I received an email from Will, a former colleague from my early days with DoD. I had not seen Will since he married and left Dallas to pursue a Ph.D. in divinity at Harvard – ten years earlier.

When I met Will in the mid-1980's, our mutual employer had begun experimenting with the construction of light reconnaissance aircraft. These one-man hang gliders powered by a small engine could be folded up and placed in the back of a pickup truck. They could be launched anywhere without the support of a formal runway. The program was the pilot for today's drone reconnaissance/strike force.

Will was a graduate of the U.S. Naval Test Pilot School (NAVAIR), and had been a test pilot for the Marine Corps. Although I did not work directly with him, we both held high profile positions with the company. I built a reputation as the leading process & logistics engineer, while Will made his reputation in project engineering as the company's chief test pilot. Will was the personification of Marvel comics' Captain America. Physically he was a blend of Troy Donahue and John Cena – only he was a compact 5'6" frame. His uniforms and business suits were always pressed razor-sharp and his blonde, buzz cut hairstyle was purposefully grown longer on top to let the hair sweep slightly across his forehead. He sported perfect, fence-post teeth that gleamed when he smiled. His personality was as commanding as I could imagine Gen. MacArthur's had been, leading the troops on the D-Day invasion. The women encouraged rumors of having dated him, and the guys secretly wanted to emulate him. As charismatic as he appeared, Will, too, was one of the "sad young men" – a fact that would take him down a dark rabbit hole.

I got to know Will in 1989 – after I left the company – when, to my great surprise, he looked me up, wanting to hang out after work and on weekends. He would drive up in this four wheel drive pickup truck that looked like it should be competing in a demolition derby, except it was adorned with a desert camouflage paint job and was immaculately maintained. Swinging a six pack of beer he would knock on my door, invite himself in and proceed to talk for hours. Sometimes he would fall asleep on my sofa for about an hour, exhausted from his ADHD, his manic personality, or his extensive daily workouts in the gym. There was no predictable schedule for these visits, but towards the end of 1991 he preferred to nap with his head resting in my lap. I recognized this need for physical closeness to be rooted in loneliness – similar to what I observed with Tony, years earlier. It was intoxicating to have this macho, boy-next-door specimen display such quiet tenderness towards me. He left suddenly for Cambridge, and I had not heard from him for a decade when I received his email.

I was scheduled to fly home that weekend, but I was curious to learn what happened to Will. So I rerouted my return flights through Miami where he had relocated to care for his ill mother. By the time my flight from London arrived in Miami it was late afternoon, and I was exhausted from travel and mentally drained from my work during the prior week. I was also recovering from the recent transition of having left Silicon Valley to join this new enterprise. I booked a suite at a Miami resort, rented a car and drove to pick up Will at his mother's house. As he got in the car, he flashed that familiar smile showing of the same over-the-top personality I remembered from the previous decade. I noticed the fine stress lines at the corners of his eyes. Will was in his mid to late fifties. Although I had no firsthand knowledge of the wild parties back in the early 1980's, in that moment, I could believe the rumors as I observed his slightly burnt-out appearance. We went to dinner and reminisced about our careers and returned to my suite with two six packs of beer. We sat on the lanai and killed off one of the six packs, catching up on our experiences during our years apart. It was not clear what Will had decided to do with his divinity studies, but I did learn that his wife divorced him several years earlier.

Around midnight, Will got up to retrieve two beers from the second six pack. He set the beer next to me, and asked if I wanted to join him. I looked up to find him holding a spoon and a syringe. I was startled at the casual nature with which he invited me to partake in whatever concoction he cooked up in that spoon, but I graciously declined, remembering the rumors about those wild parties. Although there was really no stigma attached to cocaine use, I was not a participant – I didn't even know where to buy the stuff.

And that's where the story gets weird. I really don't remember how the night ended. I woke up the next morning in one of the double beds, not knowing how I got there. Will was fast asleep on the other bed. I had a flight to catch at noon that Sunday, so I woke him up after I showered and dressed. I drove him back to his mother's house and headed out for the airport. On my way, I stopped at a service station to fill the rented car with gas, but when I pulled out my wallet I discovered my debit card was missing. I searched my luggage without success, and immediately called my bank to cancel the missing card. The bank assured me I could pick up a new one the next day. Fortunately, I could wait until then. Upon retrieving the new card, I confirmed no funds had been withdrawn during the previous 24 hours. I considered myself fortunate, and forgot about the entire incident.

At least I forgot about it until Christmas Eve day 2015 when Dr. Agha began questioning me about my drug use and sexual habits. I was completely baffled, knowing I had not been in a relationship since my time with Tony in 1983. During the first week of January I followed up with Dr. Chowdhury, and was trying to recall how I may have been exposed to the HIV, hepatitis-B, and syphilis. While talking to Dr. Chowdhury about my sexual habits (or lack thereof), I suddenly remembered the blank spaces of that Saturday evening in 2001. Surprisingly, the timeline fit the 15-year period during which the viruses had been in my body, attacking my kidneys. As I attempted to relay to Dr. Chowdhury my newfound suspicions, I realized I may have been slipped drugs that evening. This was a reasonable explanation because I could not remember anything that happened after he offered me that last beer. The blackout was complete – a total loss of consciousness and memory. My suspicion is that subsequent beers I may have consumed could have been spiked, and somehow, whatever was in Will's syringe found its way into my bloodstream.

Initially, my nephrologist and my infectious disease doctors suspected my viral infections were the result of habitual drug use and/or frequent unsafe sexual encounters. This is perfectly understandable, since the combination of HIV, hepatitis B, and syphilis are typical infections carried by habitual intravenous drug users.

However, within 30 days of initiating the anti-viral drug therapy, my HIV and hepatitis B viral loads became undetectable – a result that is not normally attained until at least 6 – 12 months of consistent treatment. As well, the syphilis was determined to have been "dead" in my system, but the 6 weeks penicillin injections were conducted as a precautionary measure. My extremely low viral loads, the speed with which the anti-viral therapies rendered the HIV and hepatitis B "undetectable", and the dead syphilis supported my contention that I was neither a drug user nor was I one who engaged in risky sexual behaviors.

I cannot prove my suspicions, but Dr. Chowdhury confirmed this scenario could have exposed me to the viruses. Perhaps the most troubling aspect of this epiphany was the fact that I had so easily suppressed the entire memory. How was this possible?

Dr. Chowdhury commented that apparently I had structured my life rigidly with a predictable set of behaviors from which I rarely deviated. I was so accustomed to living within these strictures that it was challenging for me to focus on any behaviors falling occasionally outside those parameters. The one nagging aspect of that Florida reunion is the fact that the missing bank card was never compromised. When I initially relayed my suspicions to Dr. Chowdhury I doubted my own words – until I realized it was plausible that Will had been self-medicating his PTSD even before his discharge from the Marine Corp, continuing throughout his professional life. His pathology would have been to seize an opportunity to support his drug addiction – and my blackout provided a perfect occasion to take the card. But evidently Will made no attempt to withdraw money from my account, steal my identity, or "sell" my bank card for drugs. Even though he could not resist the temptation to take the card, his inability to use it was due, I believe, to his deep-seated connection to those afternoons and evenings a decade earlier, when he would seek solace, napping curled up next to me on my sofa. He simply couldn't injure me in that way. And yet, I could have been mortally wounded by his actions – truly a cognitive dissonance.

There was no point in trying to contact Will to confirm my suspicions, because the trail had gone dark for 15 years. He would be nearing 70 today, if indeed he was still alive.

12 Revelation

I was abandoned on earth as an infant, and my tracking device had not been activated; I didn't know who my 'people' truly were or from what universe they hailed ... I don't understand Earth people, and to avoid explaining I come from another planet, I keep my head down and just try to blend in.

This quirky little narrative describes aptly how foreign human behavior can be under the microscope of my observation. My emotional and social immaturity have contributed substantively to my sense of intellectual isolation. Add my taboos to the mix, and the result is that I have been fumbling through day-to-day existence instead of truly living.

All things considered, I would not have chosen this existence. I am fascinated by the Hebrew notion of "The Guf"[19]. In Jewish mysticism the Chamber of Guf is the Treasury of Souls located in the Seventh Heaven. If I had been consulted prior to my conception, I would have voted to remain in The Guf and avoid the silent pain of earthly existence. But, alas, I was not consulted. So here I am and here I shall remain. Most of my life experience has been like watching a black and white silent film without the benefit of a musical score, subtitles or lip reading skills. There have been stolen moments of joy and, dare I say, exquisite moments that played out in vivid Technicolor® and Dolby Digital 5.1 surround sound, but these have been only a few frames sprinkled among reels of film lying on the editor's cutting room floor. I have lived most of my life with the pain of social isolation, only pretending to be a part of society.

The cognitive dissonance of my life's journey has grossly complicated my ability to settle on prescriptions and conclusions vis a vis my medical trauma. This is especially true when I consider my natural tendency to seek and then define the threads of order woven into the tapestry of entropy and chaos. As suggested by my Myers-Briggs INTJ personality profile, I tend to believe that with effort, intelligence, and consideration, nothing is impossible. And yet the engineer-scientist within me readily acknowledges that scientific discovery and evolution are triggered by unpredictable, discontiguous, and disruptive events – the framework of entropy and chaos. These contradictions make sense to me, but do not quell the angst created by my cognitive dissonance.

When I say I have merely been fumbling through day-to-day existence, I am referring to my struggle to appreciate the emotionally driven experiences of the society in which I find myself trapped. For example, I am baffled by: the

---

[19] According to Jewish mythology, in the Garden of Eden there is a Tree of life or the "Tree of Souls," that blossoms and produces new souls, which fall into the Guf, the "Treasury of Souls." Gabriel (the messenger of God) reaches into the treasury and takes out the first soul that comes into his hand. Then Lailah, the Angel of Conception, watches over the embryo until it is born.

extravagant princess-themed rituals called weddings, which cost five or six figures, and have little to do with a successful union; the mania surrounding professional sports, including memorizing the statistical minutia of players and teams, the heated debates over which team or player is better, sports-driven office pools, and online gambling; yard signs urging, *"DRIVE LIKE YOUR KIDS LIVE HERE"*, as I must continuously remind myself they caution a driver to slow down, since, to my way of thinking, I should continue at the posted speed limit because my children would not be allowed to play in the street; the romantic comedy genre of film; why 10-15% of the American population live vicariously through 20+ soap operas, daily talk shows, and "infotainment" news. (*Judge Judy* alone has a daily viewing audience of 9.9 million.) What insight for living or managing one's life could possibly be gleaned from such voyeurism?

I do not understand any of this. I wear my best poker face when I find myself trapped in polite company where such indulgences and social distractions are recounted or lived out.

I mentioned in the previous chapter my consistent inability to understand the art of flirting, which is akin to hinting, and rooted in symbolism. The fault here is not mine alone. I grew up in an environment of literal communication. My parents and those adults who influenced my early childhood were very careful and precise in their use of language. They said what they meant, and they meant exactly what they said. There was never a need to read between the lines. I laugh when I think of how radical I must have seemed to most people who encountered me during my early years. I did not understand the concept of doublespeak, and held everyone accountable for exactly what they said. I did not appreciate that people often said things for effect, e.g., to push someone's buttons or to mask true intent. I believed adults had the responsibility to speak in literal terms.

Not understanding or appreciating doublespeak as a child, I was very unforgiving.

Naturally, my literal mind was a breeding ground for distrust and suspicion. I would not discover the art of nuanced language until well into my college years. Prior to that time, I did not recognize flirtatious speech, body language, or social manipulation. I was unaware that this form of communication was a normal way to test the waters of a potential relationship. I imposed austerity upon polite conversation. Who knows how many advances I spurned due to my ignorance and naïveté? I believe this explains why I struggled to understand the lyrics to popular songs. The plausibility of the inane subtexts and expressions of often unfounded and unconfirmed longing baffled me. Misinterpretations stymied any hope of developing an appreciation for figurative prose and poetry. In this sense my life was very much two-dimensional.

Since the age of 13 I knew I did not wish to father children. It seemed cruel to intentionally bring another human being into the world. Although living in social isolation throughout my childhood was not enjoyable for me, this was my norm. As I shared previously, I was never invited to parties or celebrations in the Waterloo community. My parents never threw birthday parties for me. I celebrated my birthday with my parents and my godparents almost exclusively. At best, my parents would take me out for a dinner in my honor.

SEXUAL ORIENTATION

My unfortunate experience with Val (the girl who duped my high school community into believing I had abused an alleged relationship with her) established my deep distrust of women. Only within the last decade have I been able to enjoy the company of women in general. There have been a handful of women in my life whom I considered to be very good friends, but only in recent years have I been able to appreciate the unique sensitivity and sensuality of the women in my life.

When I entered college I observed my peer group dating and marrying. Only on rare occasions did these partnerships appear wholesome. I tried to discern intellectually what spurred the attraction. I had only three best friends throughout high school – Roger, Alan and Juanita. Upon his college graduation, Alan called (I was still enrolled at UT-Austin) and asked me to be his best man. He actually said, "I've finished college, I accepted a job at John Deere tractor works, and I bought a trailer to live in. I guess it's time to get a wife." Of course, I agreed to be his best man, but I did not understand his matter-of-fact capitulation. I flew back to Iowa and met his bride-to-be. Roger, Juanita, and I did not understand what possible advantage Alan's fiancé could imbue in his life. He married anyway, and they now have four grown children and a posse of grandchildren. I guess Alan was and remains happy. I've attended many weddings over the years, but the festivities have not engendered pangs of desire in me to partake in matrimonial bliss.

Although this book represents the first time I have publicly shared the chronology of my personal relationships, I am in no way embarrassed to talk about this aspect of my journey. However, the details of my story (1975 – 2001) don't fit nicely in casual conversation. Through the process of writing this memoir I have been astonished to learn of the interest both strangers and longtime associates have expressed in my sexual orientation. Their curiosity seems a bit odd to me because I have no such curiosity about them. However, I acknowledge that for some it is crucial to categorize my orientation. I have tried (and failed) to explain that I live life asexually. It bears repeating that I do not struggle with gender identity; I see myself as a healthy man who is comfortable with my masculinity. I view asexuality as the low or absent desire for sexual activity or the lack of sexual attraction to anyone. Certainly I have been curious about the diaspora of sexual orientation, but most of my experiences have been accidental or clumsy, at best. My taboos about sexual prowess have limited associating sex with feelings of euphoria. That is not to say that I do not appreciate beauty or attractiveness in women and men – quite the contrary. I acknowledge good looks among a miniscule portion of the population. I do not, however, seek this attractiveness nor do I respond necessarily with lust. I believe my asexuality may also be characterized as the lack of devotion to a particular sexual orientation. Yet the majority of men or women with whom I have ever discussed sexual orientation consider this to be a zero sum game; one's sexual orientation must fit exclusively into one and only one category. For me, sexual orientation is more nuanced than that. I also believe labeling may obfuscate accurate conclusions about how a person sexually interacts within society. But my opinion is definitely a minority view, and that is okay.

That said, in describing my interpersonal and sexual interactions I purposely did not ever use the word "love." This term is tossed around in our daily conversations and its use would be inappropriate on its face. The casual reader may argue these stories are metaphors for my pursuit of romance, but romance had nothing to do with my latent sexual experiences. Although I would agree that collectively these involvements did broaden my perception of sexuality. And yes, within 20 years of these encounters I did note the evolving attitudes regarding gay lifestyles, but this academic voyeurism did not intimidate or challenge my sexuality identity. I concluded that the gay community was plagued by the same emotional traumas "enjoyed" by the straight community. It was facetiously amusing to observe the gay community striving for equal rights, marriage equality, and by inference, the right to struggle with infidelity, adultery, and the mating dance in general – all equally driven by irrational emotional triggers. Neither the gay nor straight community represents a blissful advantage over the other – at least not in my eyes. Thus, my intellection has offered little clarity about romance or belonging.

As sophisticated as we would like to think our society to be, the ancient Greeks, I believe, embraced a superior understanding of sexuality and love. They spurned the notion of "romantic love" (the quest for life partnership) in favor of a more intricate understanding. Perhaps this was due to the relatively short lifespan of many in Greek society due to wars, disease and the difficulty of travel. The ancient Greeks recognized and embraced six kinds of affection.

Eros denotes sexual passion and desire (named after the Greek god of fertility).

Philia describes deep comradely friendship between brothers in arms who fought side-by-side on the battlefield. It was about showing loyalty to friends, sacrificing for them, as well as sharing emotions with them. (Another kind of *philia*, sometimes called "*storge*" embodies the love between parents and their children.)

Ludus or playful love may refer to the affection between children or young lovers. We live out our *ludus* when we sit around in a bar bantering and laughing with friends or when we go out dancing.

Agape or love for everyone was the most radical kind of love. It represents selfless love that is extended to all people, whether family members or distant strangers.

Pragma is longstanding or mature love, representing the deep understanding between long-married couples. *Pragma* encourages making compromises to help the relationship work over time, and showing patience and tolerance.

The most valued level of affection is *philautia* or love of self. The idea being that love of self infers abundant love for others (as is reflected in the Buddhist-inspired concept of "self-compassion"). The clever Greeks realized there were two types of philautia. One was an unhealthy variety associated with narcissism, while the healthier version enhanced the capacity to love others.

My trysts (as recounted earlier) are easily mapped among the ancient Greek's six levels of "love." The Pepsi man encounters were most certainly rooted in *eros*. In contrast, my experience with Tony was tinged marginally with *eros*, but suffused with *philia* to a much greater degree (the daily lengthy phone calls) and *ludus* (the magic of Circus-Circus). Tony's celebration of life was steeped in *agape*, and our time together promised the attainment of *pragma*. Strangely, my fascination with the marine test pilot, Will, touched on *philia*, but elusively promised the prize of *eros*, as I contemplated the submission of the beautiful and powerful daredevil.

I embrace most the concept of *philautia*, which best approximates my concept of a "healthy self-image" (as opposed to being selfish). Although our culture overlooks such distinctions, the sophistication of the ancients' interpretation is undiminished. Given our society's propensity for crimes of passion, and divorce rates exceeding 50%, it may be prudent to adopt a more sophisticated posture when it comes to matters of the heart.

IMPATIENCE

My preference for hiding within the safety of The Guf speaks to the impatience within my *StrenghFinder* core themes. The most notable of these being: Activator® – the impatient tendency to make things happen by turning intellection into action. So many of life's dramas (and the lessons to be gleaned from them) play out over decades. I prefer my knowledge constructs to be proactive and conclusive, but alas, this is rarely how wisdom is obtained. Epiphanies are rarely the instantaneous result of an experience. And this is why I am frustrated by having been trapped in my own Odyssey to find companionship over the past 40 years. Waiting for the deep understanding and resolution of life's puzzles has been agonizing. The sluggish process of revelation far exceeded my attention span and I became agitated and bored.

The most valuable gift of my experience with undiagnosed renal failure is that I have been forced to peer deeply into my past and perform a postmortem of sorts on my life. Friendship, passion, and emotional satisfaction eluded my grasp as deftly as the viruses masked within my apparently healthy visage eluded detection for 15 years. And yet, the elusiveness of *timely* revelations should come as no surprise when I think back on a particular story my mother shared with me about her life.

After she retired from her long career as an educator, she sought new avenues to place her professional credentials in service to her community. She was asked to assist in the revitalization of the academic library at Bishop College, a notable HBCU located in Dallas. This was a chance to put to good use her M.S. degree in Library Science. My mother viewed the project with humility and considered it a great honor. As she was integrated into the team of librarians and administrators on the project, she was reintroduced to a kind old lady who had been a contemporary of Aunt Sis (her great aunt and Granny's eldest child). Nearly 50 years had passed since she saw the old woman, but their shared stories of a more challenging but exciting time forged a nostalgic bond between the two women. One day as they worked together, the old lady asked my mother why she had not married Danon Muckleroy? The old woman made note of my mother's married name: Harvey. As old ladies tend to do, the matriarch delved into a soliloquy about the importance the Muckleroys represented during the Great Depression. Evidently oil was discovered on the Muckleroy's land in East Texas, and like the Clampetts from the popular 1960's sitcom *The Beverly Hillbillies*, the oil just kept pumping. The Muckleroys became well ensconced among the Black nouveau rich. The old lady continued her prattle (ignoring mother's interjection about having married Robert Harvey in 1942), expressing her expectation my mother (Cora) and Danon would become the "it" couple of old East Texas, and wondered aloud what happened. She plowed on relentlessly with her colorful musings until, to Cora's great surprise, she paused for a moment and turned to Cora and asked, "Would you like to meet Danon? I've told him I was working with you here at Bishop. You know he's a widower now. If you like, I'd be happy to chaperone a meeting between you two. It would be so much fun to see the two of you together again." I'm certain the old lady was not suggesting some salacious rendezvous. She was merely caught up in the excitement of sharing old and familiar memories, and was completely unaware of the distress with which Cora received her words. The name *Danon Muckleroy* was suddenly unearthed after remaining buried for 50 years in a crypt of sad and difficult memories.

During her college years in the 1930's, as Granny defended her Iowa Homestead from baseless larceny charges, Cora found herself facing financial uncertainty. She opted to suspend her course work at Wiley College for one year, renewed her cosmetology license in Harrison County, Texas and began to work full time as a cosmetologist. That is how Cora came to know Mrs. Muckleroy (Danon's mother) who sported evidently a thick mane of hair similar in texture to her own.

During the Great Depression when Granny sent Cora to live with her father in Chicago, there was no money to waste on salons. Her father was not married at the time, so Mom was on her own with respect to personal care. I always knew her to be fashionable, tailored, and well "put together", as the saying goes. I had not considered how she had developed her sense of personal style; it was just the way she was. The puzzle pieces fell together when I remembered Cora studied cosmetology as a young woman living in Chicago. I also recalled my mother sitting for several hours in front of the kitchen stove on Saturdays, skillfully wielding a pressing comb and curling irons with the same expert dexterity Rembrandt might use in handling a paintbrush. She flicked water on a hot implement as she removed it from the gas burner. Sometimes she wiped the tool on a folded towel and used more water. When the water danced to her liking, she judged the tool to be at the perfect temperature to use without damaging her hair. With the benefit of a small makeup mirror perched on the stovetop, she patiently parted her hair into manageable segments, straightening first, then curling each thick swath, one after another, affecting luster and luxurious waves. She never burned her scalp, and never missed a section.

Mrs. Muckleroy came to appreciate how swiftly and painlessly Cora combed, straightened, and curled her hair, styling it with consistent perfection. Her talent endeared Cora to Mrs. Muckleroy who became her most loyal client. Eventually she introduced Cora to her fraternal twin boys. A romance sparked between Cora and Danon, one of the twins. However, the romance ended abruptly when Granny's case concluded and Cora was able to resume to her studies. It was some time before Danon discovered that Cora had returned to Wiley, since her connection with him (through his mother) was lost.

The real oil in the milk was the product of mischievous deceit conjured by a distant cousin, Zeta who was a student at Bishop College (also in Marshall). Zeta's family lived in Detroit, where they were a very influential part of black society. There was a connection between her family and my mother's uncle (Granny's son who was a Detroit attorney). Zeta was an attractive socialite with a killer figure and a fantastic wardrobe. She was the kind of girl who could credibly quip Mae West's line: *Good girls get to go to heaven, but bad girls get to go everywhere!*

 Upon returning to Wiley, Mom somehow connected with Zeta at Bishop. Zeta was a member of Delta Sigma Theta Sorority, and Mom pledged the rival group, Alpha Kappa Alpha. In those days, the AKAs were known for beautiful light-skinned women (a la Beyoncé and Halle Berry), while the Deltas were known equally for beautiful "black" or darker-skinned women. Perhaps due to their competing sorority affiliations, there was always an unspoken but friendly competition between the two young women. Zeta knew of Cora's feelings for Danon. One fateful evening, the two went out with the Muckleroy twins. The foursome were not paired off as the evening had been quickly and casually arranged. There was a rush to get to their destination. Although my mom was happy to see Danon again, they had not had an opportunity to talk before they set out. The young men sat in the front seat, discussing the politics and business aspirations. However, the conversation in the back seat took a less than genial turn. Zeta recounted exuberantly her exploits during the previous summer and suddenly extended her left hand to show off a stunning diamond engagement ring. Although she did not actually name her fiancé, Zeta implied who it was: the driver and owner of the car in which they were passengers – Danon Muckleroy. So Zeta inferred that she and Danon were a couple, and pretended to be oblivious to Cora's romantic interest in him. She goaded Mom to share in her excitement over the prospective "merger" between her own Detroit clan and the Muckleroys – two prominent and well-to-do families. Evidently Cora fell silent and did not challenge Zeta's feigned euphoria. That was the last time my mother saw Danon. She met my father in class that summer and they married upon her graduation. Of course, it turned out that Zeta was not engaged to Danon. She was simply jealous of my mother's connection with him and his family.

My office phone rang early one afternoon in 1988. It was Mom. Her normally buoyant voice was pensive, signally immediately that she was somehow troubled. I thought perhaps a family member or friend had died suddenly. However, I was rendered nearly speechless when she asked me if I thought she should allow an old friend to arrange a meeting with a lover from 50 years ago. *What? Mom is asking for my advice about the possible risks and benefits of reconnecting with a former lover? From half a century ago? How could this be?* Although I was struck by the incredible irony of the conversation, my response was logical and in many ways, predictable. Without hesitation or emotional bias, I suggested she allow the old lady to arrange a meeting. If she needed answers, then it was probably best to speak to the source of her angst.

Mom acted on my advice. A month later my office phone rang again. This time Mom shared the details of her meeting with Danon. Even more surprising was that my counsel actually bore fruit. Cora discovered Danon had always wondered why she did not speak with him during the entire night of their last fateful meeting. His attempts to locate her were foiled by Zeta's claims that she returned to Iowa to look after her grandmother. Of course none of that was true, but Danon had no reason to doubt Zeta's story. After all, she was my mother's distant cousin. Cora also learned that Danon and his wife were childless, and when she died in the early 1980's, he had no desire to remarry. Both he and Cora were unwitting victims of a scheming and jealous woman. Danon was happy to learn that my mother had enjoyed a pleasant life with her husband, my father. Danon knew of the Harvey family from Brazoria County, Texas primarily due to my paternal grandfather's travels throughout southern and eastern Texas as a presiding elder with the A.M.E. church. At long last, their false assumptions about their estrangement could be laid to rest. Danon confessed he never loved anyone – not even his devoted wife – the way he once loved my mother, Cora Franklin. Knowing the truth, they parted on friendly terms and wished each other well.

I was happy to hear Mom's dilemma ended well. I recalled the angst I experienced during those eight months of drama my senior year in high school with the Val saga. My God! I could hardly imagine my mother suppressing half a century of uncertainty. I found it even more astounding that my mother enjoyed a pleasant life with my father. They endured World War II, Waterloo, and re-establishing their careers after transitioning from Waterloo to Dallas – and they overcame all these obstacles through their own sense of *pragma*. For an instant a pang passed through me that I may never have been born had it not been for Zeta's deceitful intercession. This thought was interrupted almost before it was fully formed when my mother posited whether or not she should tell my father about her visit with Danon. I assumed for a moment her statement was rhetorical, but that could have been wishful thinking. After a brief silence my infallible logic kicked in and I suggested she follow her heart. I learned a week later that she in fact told Dad about her meeting with Danon. Furthermore, she confessed that she did not love my father when she married him in 1942 as she had loved Danon. To her amazement, Dad told her he always had known this to be so, but that he loved her and felt lucky that she was willing to share her life with him. He held no ill will toward Danon and did not feel betrayed by her true feelings. For some reason I was not surprised to learn of my father's acceptance and acknowledgment of the situation. I was stunned to think what it must have been like for Mom to carry this burden for 45 years of marriage. I am certain I could not appreciate the depth and breadth of my mother's revelation.

PHILIA REVEALED

My father's gracious perspective toward my mother in this story is relatable to a situation I encountered in the early 1980's after I relocated from Houston to Dallas. While still in Houston, I left Dow Chemical to pursue my entrepreneurial interests. As I did so, I enjoyed the support of an exceptional probate/estate attorney whom I befriended. My venture was ultimately unsuccessful, however, and I struggled financially, especially during my last year in Houston. I left the city to embark on my new career path with the DoD in Dallas, never sharing my struggles with my attorney friend. After I was comfortably established in my new career path and after I resolved the debts accumulated during my venture, I returned to Houston as a kind of fond farewell to chemical engineering. I was abandoning the field I studied in college and expected to be part of for many, many years. During that trip I had dinner with my attorney friend. It was good to see him. He listened patiently as I enthusiastically shared the triumphs of having landed firmly on my feet following my failed venture. We were enjoying an exquisite dessert over strong coffee and heavy cream when I realized he was staring intently at me. I stopped talking and met his gaze, which was intense although he did not appear to be angry. After several moments of complete silence punctuated only by the tingling of our silverware on the dessert plates, he said to me, "I'm short and not particularly good-looking. The only thing I have going for me is that I'm one of the best damned attorneys in the state. It hurts me to learn that you did not share with me the problems you were having with your business. By not asking you selfishly denied me the opportunity to do for you what I am qualified to do. Did you think I would not be interested in helping you? After all, I helped you launch your consulting practice – I believed in the projects you landed and could have ported you through the challenges and disappointments of your business partnerships. But no – you didn't trust me enough to share your misgivings with me or seek my help. Don't you understand that there is nothing you can say or do to change my perception of you? Only I reserve the right to change my opinion of you."

His words burned in my chest like a molten sword. I did not avert my gaze as he quickly reassured me that it was disappointment, not anger that provoked his words. I never considered his perspective. I was concerned only with proving to the world that I could solve my own problems.

In 1987 my father began to evidence mild signs of Alzheimer's disease. Slow thinking and occasional memory problems are common among aging persons. Our brains change as we age like the rest of our organs. However, serious memory loss or confusion may signal major changes in the way our minds work and may indicate that brain cells are failing. The most common early symptom of Alzheimer's is difficulty remembering newly learned information because Alzheimer's typically begins in the part of the brain where learning takes place. As the disease advances it leads to progressively severe symptoms. Dr. Washington, my father's PCP, warned him a decade earlier he would likely suffer this condition and suggested mental exercises to minimize the effects. Dad was in denial about any threats to his cognitive prowess and readily rejected Dr. Washington's warnings. But as he turned 70 the predictions began to manifest. At first the signs were almost undetectable. He would be driving on the freeway and find himself unable to remember where he was going. Fortunately his ability to navigate traffic at high speeds was not affected. He was not lost – he knew where he was, but he could not remember his destination. After a few anxious moments his destination would come back to him and he would continue. Occasionally he would forget scheduled events – even those that were of keen interest to him. After a brief mention of the event and the situation in which it was first discussed, he would remember. Every now and then he would drive to his office, park the car in his assigned space and unlock his office and find himself unable to remember the short drive from his home to his office. These were minor incidents, which he was unlikely to mention unless someone happened to be present when they occurred. In which case, he would pass them off has daydreaming or having too much on his plate.

The situation took a more serious turn one Thursday as I received a phone call from my mother upon returning to my office after lunch. I know it was a Thursday because I was scheduled to board a 10 p.m. Lufthansa flight that evening for a three-week trip to Germany. Mom was hysterical. I struggled considerably to calm her down and uncover the reason for her upset. I managed to get from her that she had just received in the mail a notice of foreclosure on their home. I got the name of the mortgage company and before ending the call, I assured her I would call her back within the hour. Still, I felt certain I did not have all the details because Mom's story simply did not make sense. My parents had a modest mortgage and their household income was about $15,000 per month. A foreclosure notice was inconceivable. At first I thought of cancelling my trip, but a little voice told me to wait and make a few phone calls first. In that moment I thought of my attorney friend who had given me the tongue lashing years earlier. I called his office in Houston and fortunately he answered the phone. I shared with him my mother's story, adding my suspicion and confusion over the situation. He asked my parents' ages, the name of the mortgage company and their physical address. With this information, he told me to hang up the phone and to expect a callback in a couple hours. I told him of my imminent departure and suggested that I would cancel my trip, but he assured me there was no reason to do so.

Approximately 90 minutes later, my friend called back to say he had located the private investment group in Florida that held my parents' mortgage. He explained the situation and received confirmation from the investment group that they had called the mortgage company and instructed them to cease the foreclosure. He had also wired thousands of dollars to the mortgage company to cover the payments in arrears, including fees and penalties, and had essentially refinanced the original loan at a lower interest rate. He advised me to call my mother, give her his contact information and assure her that there was no pending foreclosure. He then bid me a fond farewell and wished me much success during my trip. I hung up and immediately called Mom with the good news. I felt her extreme relief. In all their years of marriage they had never suffered a financial crisis. My mom had been in denial about my father's diminishing mental competence, but this forced her into an unambiguous and dark reality. At that time there was little emotional support in place for Alzheimer's patients and their caregivers, and health insurance did not cover such diseases. Those without the financial means could easily suffer bankruptcy under the weight of medical expenses. Although my parents had ample financial resources, there would be a substantial emotional toll on my mother. While I was still in Germany she discovered hidden in Dad's sock drawer half a dozen envelopes addressed to their mortgage company – complete with postage. Each envelope contained a signed check. When she questioned my father, he was incoherent.

Rarely is there a downside to swallowing one's pride and asking for help from the best resources available. In this instance, the best resource available to me was the probate/estate attorney in Houston. He covered all payments and fees due without collateral. Not only did he resolve the issue, he also provided an improved situation for my parents (i.e., a lower mortgage interest rate). He accomplished all this with intellectual certainty within 90 minutes of learning of the crisis. The attorney did what he knew was best in this situation. His priority was to reestablish stability for my family and me. He did all this simply because I asked for help. My friend's actions personified *philia*.

Twenty-eight years later, acting on the advice from Dr. Chowdhury, my PCP, I informed my friends and colleagues of my medical condition. It never even occurred to me to ask anyone to be a kidney donor. In fact, I was just beginning to comprehend that I was not going to die immediately, and there was a course of treatment for me, which included the possibility of transplant surgery. I was unaware that a *living* donor was an option. Despite my personal ignorance, three persons from my circle of care volunteered to be live kidney donors. They had some marginal knowledge that this was a possibility and for reasons known only to each of them, they wanted to be there for me. Their gestures along with countless other acts of kindness and emotional support completely changed my understanding of what it means to be a friend.

During the past six months I have had frequent opportunities to revisit that dinner with my attorney friend and recall his words, "By not asking, you selfishly denied me the opportunity to do for you what I am qualified to do." These words stung with each call I received from Jason, Mark and Carl volunteering to be live kidney donors. I was overwhelmed by their unselfish and sacrificial acts as I experienced the miracle of *philia*.

Although I am admittedly a slow learner, I have come to understand that throughout my life I have been sensitive to the needs, the loneliness, and occasional isolation of others. I seem to have a knack for placing people and resources in close proximity to each other based on some expressed angst or desire. This talent flies in the face of my admitted social deficits. Sometimes I do this in secret and sometimes I simply say, "You know, I should introduce you to…", "Have you considered exploring…", or "I need to take you to… ." I don't look for affirmation or pats on the back in these situations. I just do it – and amazingly the people to whom I offer these suggestions often benefit greatly in ways that I may not learn of until many years later. I am not sure whether I just have a talent for establishing a safe place for people to explore the unknown or the unresolved issues of their life, or if I have some unconscious insight into an untapped opportunity that may benefit them. Usually I do not stick around to see what may transpire, I just "know" it was the right thing to do at the time and I believe the universe will manifest a healthy transaction for the individual – providing he or she is truly ready for it. I now understand that extending my support in this way has endeared me to people through the years in ways I could never measure. This is not something I could have planned. I am only now learning the value and impact of my *philia* and the karma it has and will continue to generate. Funny – it speaks to the old adage I heard so many times from Miss Tread, "You reap what you sow."

It bears repeating that my traumatic diagnosis has afforded me the very special gift of peering deeply into my past. The more I think about the amazing people who shaped my early years, growing up in Waterloo, Iowa, the more convinced I become that they all deserve their own feature-length film. Each was a survivor. From them I leaned not only to survive, but to thrive.

With patience, I have come to terms with my cognitive dissonance and latent sexual development. The missed opportunities resulting from these personal shortcomings are part of my past; I have learned to live in the present.

I have gained an appreciation for the value and impact of my *philia,* and claim this as my gift to others that keeps on giving.

Although I am now counted among tens of millions of Americans diagnosed with a life-threatening illness or chronic condition, I remain encouraged. This is a journey-in-progress, and the outcome is not guaranteed. Still, I move forward without fear. My prognosis is encouraging, thanks, in no small measure, to my team of doctors, and other underappreciated healthcare workers who perform daily miracles. It is my responsibility to encourage *them*. It is my responsibility to remain committed to my treatment regimen. It is my responsibility to show up consistently for medical appointments on time, and demand answers. I am my own best advocate.

Perhaps there is a silver lining to my social and emotional deficits, after all.

Afterword

RIDDLE: Why do hot dogs come in packages of ten, but hotdog buns come in packages of eight?

ANSWER: Life doesn't always work out like you want, so be happy with what you have.

This quirky riddle comes from the Ethan Reiff and Cyrus Voris script for the 2003 movie, *Bulletproof Monk*. The first time I saw this screen adaptation of the underground comic book that inspired the plot, I considered the theme of the movie to be a modern-day archetype of the 1940s – 1950s B-movies of my childhood – movies that served as my private escape into a secret world of pirate ship adventures, murder mysteries, and magical realms filled with knights, sorcerers, and reluctant heroes. During my elementary school years in Iowa, Saturdays would find me sitting cross-legged in front of a black-and-white TV – my personal crystal ball, eagerly anticipating what escapades would define the afternoon.

But today the riddle speaks to me as a clever metaphor for how one resolves the conundrum between fantastical dreams and harsh realities. Allow me to explain.

The story is about a Tibetan monk who becomes a mentor to a young street kid whom he can teach to protect an ancient sacred scroll that holds the key to unlimited power. Early on, the monk poses the riddle to the scruffy, street-wise kid. In turn, the kid chides the monk, pointing out the fallacy of his "fortune-cookie philosophy." The monk explains to the kid that when he is able answer the riddle, the kid will have found his place within the universe. My great grandmother expressed a similar lesson this way: *"It's not what you want that makes you fat; it's what you get."* In other words, we tend to envision how our destiny may play out. We pen our scripts, cast our characters, and imagine ourselves triumphantly defeating dragons and saving damsels in distress. In reality, those secret plots are often sidelined by unplanned events, unintended consequences, and the constant assault by universal fault lines over which we have little or no control.

Bulletproof Monk is a metaphor of my childhood vision: escaping Iowa, attending college, working for 25 years in a lucrative job, retiring with great wealth before the age of 50, and enjoying life with a soulmate whom I would discover somewhere along the way. My reality is that I did escape Iowa. I earned two college degrees. But I never found that single lucrative job from which I could retire after 25 years of loyal service. Instead, my career charted me through several jobs in both defense and commercial industries. And I never found that soulmate. To top it all off, in hindsight I see that the last 20 years of that eclectic career path was accomplished while I was unaware that I was gravely ill.

I never found that perfect match between hotdog buns and hot dogs. Some of the buns grew stale and had to be thrown away, and the hot dogs could not be considered nourishing no matter how many onions, chili toppings, pickles, ketchup, or mustard was heaped on top. Yet, all and all, my life has indeed been exciting, satisfying, and challenging – occasionally sprinkled with stunning discoveries, magical moments, and devastating disappointments. It has been capped with surviving the slow death experience of renal failure and learning to thrive.

But which character have I been? Protagonist, villain or reluctant hero? And who have I become? Should I allow a difficult reality to sour the totality of my life experience? Hell no! Heeding the lesson of the hot dog riddle, I am learning to be happy with what I have. Renal failure, the capstone of my saga, has transformed the diminutive black-and-white TV screen into vivid, sharp focus.

Then like folded space I am transported to New Year's Day, 2017. I sit alone in my living room, struggling to make sense of the previous 12 months as memories swirl in my head like a broken gyroscope – forward, back, upside-down and inside-out – all at the same time.

A random scene appears from four months ago. I gasp audibly. I see myself sitting in my primary care physician's office, accompanied by my trusted friend, a registered nurse, who has volunteered to be my medical advocate. Also present, is a Notary Public, who is a member of my PCP's staff. We have assembled so that I can sign my Advanced Medical Directive. An ink pen is in my hand. All I must do is affix my signature on the designated line. I place the tip of the pen on the paper, but I can't remember how to sign my name. I quickly scan my cognitive awareness, which appears to be intact. However, I am unable to execute the physical motion necessary to draw my name: *Reginald M. Harvey*. I lift the pen from the paper and force my arm to move millimeters further along the line. Again, I place the tip of the pen on the paper, but my fingers ignore my command to replicate my cursive signature, a task I have dispatched perhaps a million times. The muscle memory necessary to execute this simple task is simply not there. I am experiencing a panic attack that is deeply connected to my own fears about my ultimate identity as I face this existential medical crisis. Indeed, *who am I, If I can't sign my own name? Am I really me?* Someone asks, "Are you okay?" I can hear the bewildered concern in the voice even though I don't recognize the speaker, as all my conscious will is focused on moving the tip of that pen. I hear myself say, "I cannot sign my name." Uttering those five words makes this loss of motor function real. In my mind I am questioning how I could possibly lose the ability to certify my identity. The panic manifests as a sinking feeling, like I'm descending through the tube of a huge water slide – only there is no water and no sun. It's pitch black. I close and open my eyelids in slow motion, as if intentional, deliberate blinking will reset reality. But the situation is unchanged. The Notary approaches and quietly says, "It doesn't matter what the signature you can write today may look like. I am here to witness that you, through this action, are certifying your agreement with the content of this Advanced Directive." My brain processes these words. I understand what is being said. But the statement affords no shelter or comfort for the sinking feeling I cannot escape. Obviously, my loss of grip strength and motor control is more serious than having unwittingly tapped a funny bone. I just know I have to sign this *damn* document. Shifting to Plan B, I begin to move my entire forearm as if painting my signature on the concrete slab of a building heliport. *Broad strokes, broad strokes,* I think to myself. Looking down at the paper, I see an intelligible scribble. At least I did not drop the pen. The Notary takes the pen from my hand along with the document and says, "Thanks, I'll notarize the document and log this certification." I looked down at my right hand and repeatedly attempt to make a fist. The exercise confirms I once again have regained grip strength in that hand, although the rheumatoid arthritis has slightly warped the process of smoothly curling my fingers. Regardless of the physical effort, I realize I can, in fact, form a fist. At the same time, I am resisting the idea that my persona is now being ascribed a new label:

> "P – A – T – I – E – N – T." A new identity is overshadowing *Reginald M. Harvey*, and the format of this new moniker is something sterile like:
>
> HARV-052455-H226759-Z122179
>
> [first 4 letters of surname] – [date of birth] – [case number | policy number]
>
> I reluctantly welcome what is essentially my new signature.

Several questions arise. Which moniker is more genuine – the familiar cursive legal name or this generic and clinical file designation? How do I simultaneously embody these disparate monikers? And between them, where is my identity, my dignity, and my humanity?

A few days later, with determination and practice I regained control of the micro-muscles in my hand and was once again able to write my signature. This mini crisis was only one of many to come.

Similar unanticipated assaults – especially those from an impersonal, poorly integrated healthcare system would continue to plague my life. Almost daily there was a tug-of-war between the healthcare behemoth and myself as I attempted to reclaim my identity and cling to some sense of human dignity

Early one morning I called CVS Specialty Pharmacy to refill my three antiviral medications. It was 07:36 a.m. –usually the best time of day to maneuver efficiently through the automated call options to access a pharmacy technician. But on this day the pharmacy tech informed me that my account had been placed on hold until I make a payment on my outstanding balance. I ask, "What outstanding balance?" Without emotion the pharmacy tech tells me that my account indicates I have failed to pay an outstanding balance of $1450. Remaining calm, I requested a transfer to the billing business unit, and was dispatched to a new staffer who confirmed the same past due balance. I challenged the past due amount, stating that I had been refilling the exact same three antiviral drugs since February 2016 – with no co-pay levied. The staffer restated in a monotone timbre the past due amount, ignoring my statement. So, I summoned my evil twin (my alter ego) to burst through the air of complacency. "Help me understand how less than 30 days ago when executing the same refill request, I had zero-dollar co-pay, and today you tell me my account is suspended until I pay you a past due amount of $1450? I need these drugs to stay alive. Nothing has changed with my insurer or my insurance program. Explain to me what's behind this sudden $1450." I am livid, and I can tell by the breathing of the staffer that I have successfully shattered her detached demeanor.

After an extended period of audible keyboard clicks, the staffer asks, "Mr. Harvey, when did you change your insurance plan?" Now I am even more irate, having previously stated that there have been no changes to my insurance plan or to my insurance carrier.

I challenge, "I am a corporate employee of CVS Health, and am covered by the Aetna/CVS plan that is extended to all 275,000 employees. As you are an agent of CVS Health, you know that the Aetna/CVS insurance plan is only renewed in June of each calendar year. As we are in the first quarter of 2017 (the dreaded insurance 'donut hole' of coverage) it is obvious there has been no opportunity to change my insurance plan!"

More keyboard clicks. Finally, the staffer responds, "Our records show your insurance to be with [Omnicom]. We have been billing [Omnicom] and they have been rejecting the pharmaceutical claim."

"Who in the hell is [Omnicom]? I just told you my insurance provider is Aetna/CVS."

"Well, Mr. Harvey, somehow your profile has identified your insurer to be [Omnicom]."

"I don't even have access to your database and there is no way for me to have requested any change to my profile."

"If you don't mind, sir, could you please give me the group ID and member ID on your Aetna/CVS insurance card."

Incensed, but feeling somewhat triumphant, I provide the requested group and member ID numbers. Moments later the financial staffer confirms that the pharmaceutical claim has been approved. I inquire about the status of the reported past due amount of $1450, but the staffer indicates that the past-due charge has been wiped from the system and the account hold has been rescinded. With apologies, I am transferred to yet another pharmacy tech to complete my refill transaction. Forty-five minutes have elapsed to complete a simple refill, which should have taken no more than ten minutes.

I reflect on what has just happened and shudder at the thought that neither my legal name nor my clinical file designations are sufficient protections against assaults on my identity and my sense of human dignity. *I realize that I no longer am in control here.* I think, 'Wow – the healthcare system has just hacked my identity and I am vulnerable to this happening again, without warning!

THE LIVING DONOR JOURNEY CONTINUES – KIDNEY PAIRED DONATION

About one third of people who volunteer to donate a kidney will be incompatible with their intended recipient due to blood type or human leukocyte antigen (HLA). Kidney paired donation (KPD), a kidney exchange strategy, circumvents the incompatibility between donor and intended recipient by redistributing organs among two or more donors prior to the transplants.

In the simplest type of KPD, two donors exchange kidneys so that their two candidates can each receive a compatible transplant. The donor operations are usually started simultaneously to prevent the situation in which one donor decides not to donate after that donor's intended recipient has already received a kidney.[20]

Carl, my core strength trainer, is one of seven people who threw their hats in the ring, volunteering to be tested as potential live kidney donors. Seven people cared enough about me to offer a selfless act to save my life. And they did so on their own – without a single request from me! I was amazed and I will always be grateful for each act of kindness. Unfortunately, six of six volunteers had been rejected as incompatible donors by the time Carl stepped forward.

---

[20] Montgomery RA, Zachary AA, Ratner LE, Segev DL, Hiller JM, Houp J, et al. *Clinical Results from Transplanting Incompatible Live Kidney Donor/Recipient Pairs Using Kidney Paired Donation.* JAMA. 2005; 294(13):1655–63.

An expanded version of KPD may include exchanges among three or more pairs. The donor of one pair gives the recipient of the next pair, whose donor gives to the recipient of the next pair, and so on, until the last pair's donor gives to the recipient of the first pair in the cycle. Moving to three-way or larger exchanges significantly increases the likelihood that any pair will find a match.

Many extensions to this concept, such as larger exchanges, compatible paired donation, and use of non-directed (altruistic) donors, have allowed greater numbers of people to find matches. KPD is the fastest-growing modality of living donation in the U.S., growing from just a handful of transplants in 2000 to surpass 500 transplants per year in 2010.[21] Kidney exchange accounted for nearly ten percent of living kidney transplants in 2011.

Because the National Organ Transplantation Act of 1984 forbade acquiring or transferring a kidney for valuable consideration, members of the transplant community pressed the U.S. Congress to pass the Charlie W Norwood Living Organ Donation Act of 2007, clarifying that kidney exchange was legal.

Methodist Specialty and Transplant Hospital (San Antonio) has the largest KPD program in the U.S. Using sophisticated computer software, the team provided matches to 134 patients between 2008 and 2011. Dr. Agha, the nephrologist who originally diagnosed my renal failure, is a former medical director of the San Antonio KPD program. He lobbied the current medical director to review my medical records. It was Dr. Agha's advocacy coupled with Carl's willingness to be my "directed" live donor that made my admission into this program a reality in November 2016.

With the KPD option, Carl would donate his kidney via the San Antonio facility and they in turn would match me with a perfectly compatible live kidney donor selected from the KPD registry.

Carl and I made the four-hour drive to San Antonio on Monday, December 11, 2016, for the extensive pre-surgical KPD transplant evaluation with the program's medical coordinator. The following morning at 6:30, we stood in line with half a dozen others at the Methodist

---

[21] Terasaki PI, Gjertson DW, Cecka JM. *Paired Kidney Exchange Is Not a Solution To ABO Incompatibility.* Transplantation. 1998; 65(2):291.

Specialty and Transplant Hospital, waiting for the doors to open. Registration proceeded without incident as all our paperwork aligned with the medical records electronically transferred to the San Antonio facility in advance. But just to be certain, I had packed hard copies of every document I could lay my hands on.

Carl and I were escorted to different examination theaters in the hospital. By 10 a.m. the preliminary interviews and blood draws had been completed. I received an abbreviated interview and was told that a thorough review of the records received from Dallas Methodist Health Center warranted my approval for the KPD program. This was good news. By 11 a.m. I was escorted back to the waiting room where I found Carl engaged in conversation with a middle-aged couple.

My presence was not immediately noticed, as I opted to sit quietly in an adjacent area while the couple continued their conversation with Carl. I learned that the wife underwent a kidney transplant four weeks earlier and was at the hospital for a routine follow-up examination. Holding her husband's hand, the woman explained that during the period immediately preceding her transplant, she was not responding well to dialysis, and her condition was rapidly deteriorating. She was very near death. Although her two sisters had been tested as viable donors, both refused to donate a kidney to save her life. At this point the woman began to shiver and cry silently as her husband wrapped his arms around her, rocking her gently while stroking her hair. After a while, she wiped away the tears with a crumpled Kleenex and gathered herself, sitting upright and turning slightly to face Carl. At that moment my eyes met hers, and Carl turned to follow her gaze. He got up and beckoned me over to the couple for introductions.

"This is my friend, Reggie. We came here to be evaluated as participants in the kidney paired donation program. Reggie and I have slightly mismatched blood group types, but I am his 'directed' live kidney donor."

"But you are not related?" Puzzled, the woman turned back and forth to look at her husband and then back at Carl and me.

"You have to understand," interjected the husband. "We are astounded that you would be willing to sacrifice your kidney for someone who is not a blood relative."

"Of course I would," Carl replied. "Reggie's my friend."

The husband continued, "We were struggling with the shock that my wife's sisters both refused, even after finding out they both were viable matches. It just so happened that within hours of them telling us they refused to participate in the surgery, her distant aunt just happened to call her cell phone. I answered that call, merely as a diversion from the temporary insanity of the moment and was surprised that it was my wife's aunt. She did not know anything about my wife's medical trauma, nor had anyone in the family mentioned the siblings having been tested as potential live donors. In my stupor, I succumbed to her interrogation on what was going on, and then the call ended abruptly. My wife asked who I had been speaking with, and I told her that her aunt, upon understanding the situation, had ordered us to stay here at the hospital. She had hung up the phone to catch the first flight to San Antonio. Later that day she arrived here to be tested, and miraculously she was also a match. The transplant surgery took place that evening. So, you see within half a day we went from anticipating planning her funeral to getting a second chance at life. And all that trauma was with family. And you are here voluntarily and are willing to make the sacrifice for someone not related."

"Bless you," the woman said to Carl as she took his hand in hers and squeezed it. Just then, a nurse approached and called the woman for her examination. We said farewell as the husband followed his wife through the double doors. Carl and I sat for the next five or ten minutes in silence, looking at one another and reflecting on what we had just heard. Our reverie was interrupted, as another nurse emerged through the same double doors. She walked over to Carl to inform him that the initial test results indicated he was pre-diabetic, and therefore was not a suitable candidate for the KPD program. She went on to explain that although Carl was physically fit and likely healthy, the prediabetes coupled with the family history of diabetes constituted a future risk that he could develop a medical condition that may compromise his own kidney function. That was a risk the KPD program was not willing to subject him to. She thanked us both as she dismissed us. In shock, we sat there in silence for a while. Then I noticed Carl's expression and realized he appeared to be even more traumatized by the news than I. As it was now around noon and we'd had only juice and muffins six hours earlier, I suggested we leave the hospital and get a hearty lunch. We could check back with the hospital later with any follow up questions.

I drove us to La Tuna Grill, a quaint South-Town culinary favorite among the locals, across from the Blue Star District. Carl remained silent as he followed me to our seats on the patio. I ordered an assortment of tapas to start the meal, and only after savoring those delicacies he seemed to come out of his stupor. Just then, my phone rang. It was Lauren, the medical coordinator from the hospital, calling to apologize for not coming out personally to explain the test results. Lauren confirmed that although Carl had been eliminated, I was still considered a viable participant, provided that I could find another suitable directed donor, maintain my healthy status, and my viral loads remained undetectable. I relayed Lauren's apologies and her assessment to Carl, adding, "I sense your disappointment, but please understand that it is only because of your selfless generosity to present yourself as my directed donor that I have, one, been accepted into a second transplant program, and two, have been deemed of significant character for Dr. Agha to have placed his professional reputation on the line for me with his colleagues here in San Antono. This is a triumph – even though we don't have the outcome we'd hoped for." Carl listened intently, and after a fabulous meal (the food really is exceptional), returned to his usual, jolly self.

It was time to make the journey back to Dallas.

MAINTENANCE DIALYSIS THERAPY

Dr. Agha's decades of experience, informed by his seasoned mentors, taught him not to rush into maintenance dialysis therapy. He believes there are very practical reasons to buck the standard of care in this instance. Not the least of which is: once dialysis begins, it must be continued for the natural life of the patient, barring a successful kidney transplant. Otherwise, the patient would likely succumb to chronic kidney disease.

It had been Dr. Agha's intent to transplant me before I had a medical need for maintenance dialysis therapy. However, it was now September 2017 and no viable living donor or cadaver organ had presented. I have no parents – I am an adult orphan. I have no siblings, children, nieces or nephews. At the same time, only 20 per cent of the U.S. population shares my blood type (B), further limiting a viable organ donor pool.

Dr. Agha found it necessary to prescribe dialysis treatment in September 2017, because my creatinine levels crept past 1.4mg/dl and were now measuring between 1.5 to 1.7mg/dl, indicating that my kidney function would not be sustainable much longer. Normal creatinine levels measure between 0.7and 1.3mg/dl. Dr. Agha recommended the peritoneal dialysis (PD) method for me.

MEDICARE APPLICATION PROCESS

I chose United Health Care (UHC) as my Medicare administrator because I was already a member of AARP, and UHC was a preferred AARP provider. I believed I had carefully researched my pre-transplant medication schedule with the federal system. But my naiveite did not prepare me for how the State of Texas manages the federal Medicare program. The online UHC application process for traditional Medicare (parts A and B), the Medicare Supplemental policy, and the Medicare Rx policy took eight hours to complete. I was 63 years of age when Dr. Agha prescribed the maintenance dialysis therapy. In the State of Texas, if the patient is under the age of 65, the patient is charged a monthly premium of $1,200 or $14,400 each year until that patient turns 65. My online application was converted to a hardcopy document, which was express mailed to me with a prepaid return envelope. I was instructed to sign and return the hardcopy document. Once received, my Medicare Card, Supplemental Card and Rx Prescription Drug Cards would be issued, and my coverage authorized, retroactive to February 1, 2018. When I learned of the $1200 monthly premium, I called UHC customer service to ask why, during the 8-hour application process, I had not been informed of this. The customer service agent's response was, "Mr. Harvey, do you wish to disenroll from the Medicare program?" I lost all my composure, raised my voice, and replied, *"Not unless you can fart $70K a year for my PD maintenance dialysis therapy plus another $180K out of your ass to pay for my future kidney transplant."* There was an uneasy silence. I resumed, "No. I do not wish to *disenroll*. I am saying that I would have remembered being told I would be on the hook for $14K out-of-pocket because I live in the State of Texas." Following that exchange, my application was processed, Medicare assumed 100% of the dialysis costs, and reported their intent to pay for the transplant surgery to Dallas Methodist Transplant Center – my primary registered transplant program.

PERITONEAL DIALYSIS (PD) BEGINS

In October 2017 a dialysis therapy port was implanted in my chest to accommodate the peritoneal therapy. PD ports are typically placed on the left or right side of the anterior abdominal wall, near the belly button. The outer cuff of the port is placed subcutaneously, and the skin exit site should be 2-4 cm lateral from the cuff. The skin wounds are closed with intradermal resorbable sutures. For whatever reason the surgeon performing this port implant procedure chose my exit site to be in my chest rather than nearer my groin (for hygienic reasons). I learned later from Dr. Agha that a debate had been ongoing about the efficacy of exit port locations.

Still, nothing could have prepared me for my experience at the surgical center. Once prepped and anesthetized, I remember hearing distant banging and shouting as I neared unconsciousness. I woke up in recovery to discover the procedure had been interrupted. A nurse was telling me that I would be rescheduled in several weeks for a "redo." Apparently, just as they put me under, the fire department descended on the surgery center to conduct some sort of scheduled inspection of safety and evacuation alarms. This really happened. So, the center had been forced to interrupt my procedure. Meanwhile, I was in a stupor, recovering from the anesthesia. I was in a state of confusion, and to some extent, panicky. It was several weeks before the procedure could be rescheduled.

The second time, everything went as planned. Even so, I awakened from the procedure in a complete panic! I thought I was losing my human-ness. Seeing and touching this inanimate object dangling from my chest reminded me of the *Borg Collective*. I was being assimilated into the single hive mind from Star *Trek*.

After the access port implant procedure, I was assigned to a dialysis center that would administer my maintenance dialysis care, including training, monthly labs and physicals, therapy supplies, and coordination of provisioning and monitoring the portable wi-fi enabled cycler machine. My training to perform the manual self-administered peritoneal therapy was scheduled to begin in November 2017 and lasted through January 2018.

During this period, I was placed in an isolation unit within the dialysis center for up to six hours at a time. There, I learned to clean the port line from the access point in my chest to the connector for the dialysis solutions, establishing the platform for the dialysis that would take place at night while I slept.

I learned about the bacterial infections that could occur, how to detect them, how to administer the counter medications into the dialysis platform riggings, and how (and to whom) I should report such instances.

Two to three times a week I returned to the isolation unit to practice setting up the PD platform, prepare the dialysis solutions, and connect the port from the access point in my chest to the PD platform.

In the third month, I was in the isolation chamber every other day to practice the manual, gravity-driven PD therapy before finally being released on my own.

Meanwhile, the dialysis center set up the process for monthly delivery of my dialysis fluid prescription and ancillary PD supplies (gauze, bandages, surgical tape, tubing, tube-compliant connectors, etc.). Additional supplies would be provided by the dialysis center, as needed during my monthly clinical lab draws and nephrologist consults.

I rallied my PCP and my friends as an emergency action team to support me through the daily PD maintenance dialysis therapy and monthly restocking of supplies. I installed two seven-foot storage cabinets in my bedroom where my housekeeper stored the monthly delivery of 50 cases of supplies.

In April 2018 a new, portable wi-fi enabled cycler machines (estimated cost, $24,000) replaced the old gravity-fed, manual rigging.

The estimated $70,000 annual cost of my maintenance dialysis therapy was covered by Medicare.

To the shock of the dialysis center training nurse and staff, I never suffered any issues with peritonitis or other typical infections. I told them at the beginning of training (November 2017) that I was not going to suffer any complications. I expressed being grateful for the training and expense necessary to help me through the process, but that I truthfully wished I had never met any of them. Therefore, I would diligently follow their express instructions regarding hygiene, sanitation, preparation, cleanup, and the routine execution of the peritoneal treatment process. Therefore, should complications arise it would not be attributable to a failure of due diligence on my part. I explained that I didn't want to be there in the first place, but since I was, I *damn sure* wasn't going to commit any errors requiring emergency interventions. At first, they thought I was delirious. But the monthly clinical lab results proved that my predictions were spot on! Eventually the staff and doctors caught on to my gallows humor and attention to detail. I am extremely grateful that I never had to deal with any bacterial infections during those 26 months of PD maintenance therapy.

***

For the next 26 months I remained on call with my hospital go-bag ready, mobile phone always charged, and gas tank full, prepared for the call from United Network for Organ Sharing (UNOS)[22], announcing availability of a cadaver kidney that was a perfect match to my DNA/RNA profile.

Upon receiving such a call, the recipient has only 60 minutes to call back and acknowledge the notification, and six hours to report in person to their registered transplant center. Unless both requirements are met, the prospective recipient forfeits their placement on the UNOS list, and the organ is awarded to the next prospect on the list. The rationale for these strict rules is apparent: with the death of a donor the clock begins to tick. The process of tissue death, plus harvesting, testing, matching, and shipping make this process extremely time sensitive. Ideally, a transplant must take place within 12 hours, but no more than 24 hours at the extreme.

The traumatic experiences continued during this period. It is still hard for me to believe that I received three calls – three false alarms -- notifying me that a possibly viable, matching kidney had been identified, was available, and was being offered to me. It is important to

---

[22] United Network for Organ Sharing (UNOS): www.unos.org

note that before heading to the hospital, I was required to pack up the PD cycler device in its travelling case and bring it with me, just in case a dialysis therapy session was necessary in the hospital prior to the transplant surgery. It was my understanding that bringing my device would mitigate any shortage of equipment at the hospital:

First offer: Between 8:15 a.m. - 8:30 a.m. Wednesday, October 10, 2018, I received a call from Dr. Agha, indicating that a kidney was being offered and I had first right of refusal. At the time I was coming down from nitrous oxide and Novocain, following a dental procedure. The organ was from a 63-year-old diabetic, and the useful life was estimated to be eight to ten years. Offer declined.

Second Offer: About five months later, just after hooking myself up to the PD maintenance treatment system around 9 p.m., I received a call from the Methodist Transplant Center RNA lab that I should stop my treatment and prepare to leave for the hospital. Evidently, another prospective organ was being tested. I would receive another call within the hour to confirm. I stopped the dialysis cycler machine, disconnected the device from the dialectic fluids and disconnected myself from the cycler. I packed the cycler device into its travel case, got dressed, and lay in bed, waiting for the confirmation call. The call came, but the organ was not a viable match to my DNA/RNA profile. False Alarm.

Third Offer: On a Friday in November/2019 I received another call from the Methodist Transplant Center RNA lab that another kidney had been identified as a prospective match for me. I started the packing sequence while awaiting the confirmation call. I loaded the PD cycler device in the trunk of my car beside my "go" bag. I went back inside to wait for the call. Once again, the "match" was determined not viable. False alarm.

However, this time there was a twist in the back story. The next day I called Dr. Agha's office to ask what was going on. A few hours later, Dr. Agha returned my call and explained that the call from the RNA lab had been prompted by my DNA/RNA profile on file. (NOTE: Every quarter special blood panels would be drawn and sent to the RNA lab to track any shifts in my blood profile). However, the RNA lab had indeed written a revised DNA/RNA profile on a Wednesday of that week but did not publish the change to the UNOS system until the following Monday. Therefore, the notice I received Friday was based on my old profile. Per safety protocols the unpublished revision to my DNA/RNA profile was discovered and subsequently the match had been canceled. Upon hearing this, I was numb more than angry or frustrated. I explained to Dr. Agha that in the scientific/engineering environment that was part of my professional orientation, the RNA lab would have set an "effective date" so that all parties could have intellectual certainty about the timing of activating the new profile. Had that been done, I would not have been subjected to the inconvenience and trauma caused by an erroneous notification. He apologized, saying he would share my recommendation with the team.

On December 15, 2019, the Methodist Transplant Center informed me in writing that stabilized changes in my blood titres (*the concentration of an antibody, as determined by finding the highest dilution at which it is still able to cause agglutination of the antigen*) allowed me to receive a kidney of blood type A or B, significantly expanding my donor pool.

The Transplant Event Arrives | "Day **One**" – Second Birthday

By now I have become numb to the psychological trauma caused by errant notifications. Ironically, on April 15, 2020, at about 9:30 a.m., I happened to be at the Methodist Dallas Transplant Center filling out forms when the final UNOS notification arrived. The transplant center staff went into a frenetic mode verifying my whereabouts. Some staff knew I was scheduled to be at the Transplant Center that day. I answered my mobile phone and immediately notified the team with whom I was working that the UNOS call had just come through, and that I was the person everyone was frantically trying to locate. The mood at the Center switched from frenetic to euphoric! Everyone was coming to me to assess my level of excitement. To most people's amazement I remained dispassionate. While I was grateful that a transplant *seemed* eminent, due to the prior errant notices, I adopted a wait-and-see attitude.

The Covid-19 nation-wide shutdown, initiated in March 2020, causing hospitals and medical centers to suspend elective surgeries to (1) preserve available bedspace for the meteoric rise in Covid patient admittance, and (2) to isolate visitors and extraneous personnel from medical campuses. The patient isolation process enacted by Methodist Transplant Center worked in my favor:

The Center isolated non-Covid patients to the fifth through ninth floors. All other cases were limited to the first through fourth floors. Nurses assigned to Covid treatment were rotated off-duty after two weeks, sent home for a week, tested for Covid twice, and then reassigned to non-Covid duty. The same process applied to nurses assigned to non-Covid care. This process resulted in more staff available to care for patients like me. I was in heaven.

I was formally admitted to the Methodist Transplant Center that same afternoon and told that my transplant was scheduled for 4 p.m. The surgery would take about four hours. However, 4:00pm came and went. 4:15 p.m. came and went. 4:30 p.m. came and went.

Finally, I was told the surgery had been rescheduled for "later that evening." Due to the emotional trauma of the prior false notifications, I remained both skeptical and ambivalent. At 8:00 p.m. a team of people invaded my room, transferred me to an operating room bed, gave me an antiseptic sponge bath, shaved the appropriate surgical areas of my abdomen, wrapped me in blankets, and wheeled me through hallways and several service elevators to a frigid operating room. I felt disoriented but a sliver of hope began to crack my hardened emotional shell. I heard someone summarizing what was about to take place and asking me if I understood where I was and what was happening. Then the anesthesiologist introduced himself and asked me to count backwards.

I began, "100, 99,98... 97... 97..."

I awoke violently, feeling like I was floating, with no concept of how much time had passed. I felt like I was doing cartwheels before several hands grabbed my ankles and upper shoulders. All I could see was a an extremely bright, blue-white light. Now I felt as though I were free-falling, and the hands were pushing me down in mid-space. Several distant voices seemed to be speaking over one another. Abruptly the spinning and cartwheels stopped. I lay still, supported by a bed. Now I could see the operating room, and slowly my memory began to return as a voice said, "You are okay. You are safe." I have no idea how long I was in the operating room, but "soon" after the traumatic awakening a small team wheeled me back to my room. (I later learned I had been returned to my room at around 2a.m.). I was unaware that a catheter had been inserted into my penis. I was sufficiently lucid to ask the nurse what was happening. I recall that she seemed uncharacteristically giddy. I pushed further, and she explained that every hour since returning from the transplant surgery that the catheter bag proved I was urinating (on average) some 790ml of fluid every hour. To provide context, prior to the transplant I barely produced 100ml of fluid per day. The nurse explained that they would be monitoring the catheter until there was no more blood in the urine collected. (It would be another 24 hours before blood was imperceptible).

Around 10 a.m., I heard a professional but heated discussion outside my door. Eventually, I learned that the debate had been between the surgeon who supervised the transplant (whom I had consulted several times in the months before) and the nephrologist (a member of Dr. Agha's team, charged with supervising my post-transplant recovery). The debate was about how soon to consider removing my PD maintenance port. The transplant surgeon preferred to leave the port implanted for at least a week, until he was certain the transplanted kidney was stable and reliably performing. The nephrologist insisted that the port be removed within the next 24 hours. Finally, the nephrologist stated, "You are a brilliant surgeon, and your work was stellar. You've completed your job. Mr. Harvey is my patient, and I will determine when the port is removed – not you." With that said, the door to my hospital room swung open and this petite, 5'2" person entered the room. I chuckled silently, visualizing the hallway debate, as the surgeon was 6'7". But there was no debate as to who the alpha personality was. The very next day I was once again in an operating room as my BORG days finally came to an end. The port was gone. No more tubes. I was elated!

A LITTLE HELP FROM MY FRIENDS

It was back in December 2015 when Dr. Agha informed me that I "could have gone to sleep and never awakened." Only then did I discover that during the preceding months and years, I had been blithely living a slow death experience, completely unaware of my grave medical condition.

After a long, arduous journey, including two years of daily peritoneal dialysis therapy, I was successfully transplanted on April 15, 2020 – AKA my second birthday. The only thing I know about the donor is that he was an athletic, 27-year-old male.

I had assembled a transplant response team, a subset of the persons in my circle of my care, but as it turned out, they were not needed. My longtime friends Mark and Tina, a couple I first met in 1996, "kidnapped" me from the hospital upon my discharge, informing me that for the next thirty days, I would be staying with them. No one from my transplant response team objected, and that was that.

My time in Mark and Tina's care was a period of many intricate adjustments, too many to be recounted here. With effort, I suppressed the micro-manager that is native to my persona, and relinquish control to my hosts. Mark drove me to my frequent consults with the post-transplant medical team.

I lost 50 pounds of accumulated "fluid" weight, a by-product of peritoneal dialysis. I retrained my bladder so that it functioned seamlessly with my digestion – truly a bizarre mind/body exercise. During this period, I was most vulnerable to bacterial infections, because my immune system had been intentionally destroyed to reduce the possibility that the new kidney might be rejected. I am pleased to report I suffered no bacterial infections. Furthermore, there was no need to put me on a restricted diet or fluid intake program.

My smooth recovery is due in no small measure to Mark and Tina's generosity. Their amazing gift freed me from the burden and distraction of organizing food deliveries, pharmacy visits, and driving myself to and from the Transplant Center. I was able to concentrate on allowing my body to recover, and regaining my strength.

I must admit that for a time I struggled psychologically to give up the peritoneal dialysis routine, which had been a required ritual every evening for two years. There was no margin of error in that tedious procedure, which was indispensable for my survival. But eventually I was able to let it go.

And it was no small feat to adjust to the reality that after nearly five years, I was no longer in limbo, waiting and wondering how my saga would turn.

Today, the transformation is complete. My slow-death journey is behind me as I welcome the experience of life lived with a truly manageable chronic condition.

No, you don't always get what you want in life. But sometimes you come really, really close.

Thank you, to my medical team. Thank you, to my circle of care. Thank you, Carl. Thank you, Mark and Tina!

ABOUT THE AUTHORS

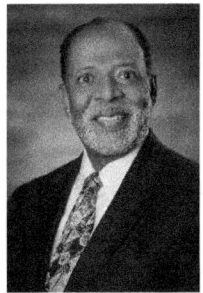

Reginald Harvey is an intelligent and well-spoken survivor with a lot to say. His medical trauma, penchant for storytelling, and expertise in manufacturing processes qualify him uniquely to write this book.

Harvey earned a B.S. in Business Management from LeTourneau University and an M.S. in Science and Technology Commercialization from the University of Texas at Austin. As a subject matter expert in business operations and product engineering logistics, he contributed to substantial performance improvements and project values across a spectrum of clients, including CVS Health, Boeing Defense & Space, and the North Atlantic Treaty Organization (NATO).

Harvey grew up in Waterloo, Iowa, a modest midwestern farming community in the 1950's and 60's. On the surface the environment was uncomplicated and nurturing. However, as college-educated professionals, his parents were essentially misfits, which rendered Harvey and his sister misfits as well. Feeling alone in a community of 85,000, Harvey learned to be fiercely independent, a trait he carried into his professional life, and was the foundation for his public persona – that is, until his medical diagnosis in 2015.

As Harvey began his medical odyssey, his primary care physician recommended journaling as a potentially healing activity. Indeed, it was in the act of writing about his experience that Harvey leaned to lay aside his invincible public image and embrace his authentic self – with all his vulnerabilities – and appreciate his talents and flaws alike.

Harvey lives in Dallas and works part-time as a consultant with Three Owls Data and Distribution Inc.

Joy Strickland is a freelance writer, ghostwriter, and editor. Her essays have appeared on HuffPost.com, CNN.com, DallasNews,com, and other media. She is also a certified wellness coach who promotes health and wellness on her YouTube channel @2BWell.

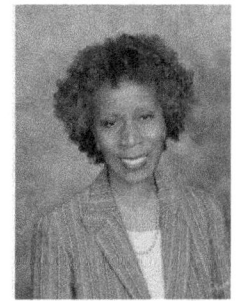

A former nonprofit executive, Strickland published *Joy in the Morning – A Mother's Journey from Tragedy to Triumph* (2010) to share the organization's origin story. In a terrible, random crime, Strickland's older son and his friend were abducted and killed by two drug-crazed teenagers. At the behest of her two friends – an attorney and a Justice of the Peace – Strickland co-founded Mothers Against Teen Violence (MATV), leading the organization for two decades. Her advocacy for violence prevention and drug policy reform earned a bevy of awards and was highlighted by: CNN and CNN *Headline News*; *USA Today*; USA Radio; *Dallas Morning News,* and other media.

A former IBM marketing executive, Strickland earned a B.S. in Mathematics from the University of Texas at Austin.

Strickland lives in Dallas with husband Greg Mahnesmith.

www.ingramcontent.com/pod-product-compliance
Lightning Source LLC
Chambersburg PA
CBHW062100220526
45471CB00010B/3551